PUTTING OUT THE FIRE

PUTTING OUT THE FIRE

New Hope for RSD/CRPS

Dr. Katinka van der Merwe

Copyright © 2016 Dr. Katinka van der Merwe
All rights reserved.

ISBN-13: 9781534832640
ISBN-10: 1534832645

This book is dedicated to the following people:

To my best friend and husband, Kevin, who saw my passion the very first time he saw me and loved me for it.

Disclaimer

The information written in this book is designed to provide helpful information on RSD/CRPS and the subjects discussed. This book is not meant to be used to diagnose or treat any medical condition or to replace the advice of your physician(s). The author of this book does not claim to have found a cure for RSD/CRPS or any other specific condition. The author of this book treats the central nervous system only, often resulting in the body being able to heal itself.

The reader should regularly consult a physician in matters relating to his or her health, particularly with respect to any symptoms that may require diagnosis or medical attention. For diagnosis or treatment of any medical problem, consult your own physician(s).

The publisher and author are not responsible or liable for any damages or negative consequences from any treatment, action, application, or preparation to any person reading or following the information in this book. References are provided for informational purposes only and do not constitute endorsement of any websites or other sources. Readers should be aware that the websites listed in this book might change.

A small body of determined spirits fired by an unquenchable faith in their mission can alter the course of history.

—MOHANDAS (MAHATMA) GANDHI

Contents

Foreword······································· xix
My Story······································ xxiii

Chapter 1 The Basics: Understanding the Nature of the Monster······1
Tracing the Monster's Footprints through History··········2
Deconstructing the Monster··························5
The Roll of the Genetic Dice: Is CRPS Hereditary?··········8

Chapter 2 The Bad and the Ugly: Mysterious Symptoms You May Not Associate with CRPS······················13
The Well-Known Symptoms························15
Your Cranial Nerves: The Front Door to Your Nervous System··································16
Your Achy Head and Neck·························18
Burden on Your Shoulders························19
Midback and Chest·····························20
Low Back····································20
Abdomen (when you are passing more gas than a pregnant woman expecting triplets)·················21
Hips/Legs/Feet (Honey, no one is running a marathon around here anytime soon.)······················21
All the Other Icky Symptoms······················22

Chapter 3 You Are Not an Island: How CRPS Affects the Lives of Those Around You···························25
You Did Not Choose This························26

	The Day the Music Dies: CRPS (AKA the Suicide Disease)··28
	Loving Someone Who Suffers from CRPS: What It's Like to Feel Like Collateral Damage·················29
	Heartbreak at Its Worst: When You Aren't Able to Be the Parent You Want to Be ·················32
	The Horror of Watching the Monster Attack Your Child ···34
Chapter 4	The Perfect Storm: How You Got Sick ············38
	Mechanistic versus Vitalistic Approaches to Symptom Treating and Healing ···················39
	The Mechanistic View················39
	The Vitalistic View···············41
	Your Amazing Body ··················42
	That Overused Word: Stress·············44
	Physical Stress·················45
	Chemical Stress ···············47
	Diet Sugars: Just Go for the Sugar if You Must ·········48
	What Is Aspartame Made Of? ··············49
	Aspartic Acid (40 Percent of Aspartame) ··········49
	How Aspartate (and Glutamate) Cause Damage ········49
	Cosmetics···················50
	Emotional Stress················52
	Emotional Stress and How It Affects Your Nervous System ··52
	So How Does One Avoid…Life?············55
	Step 1: Make the Link ··············56
	Step 2: Quit Acting Like an Ostrich ···········56
	Step 3: Neutralize the Acid·············57
	Step 4: Selfishly Forgive Others ············58
	Step 5: Forgive Yourself ··············59
	Lying in Wait: The Makings of a Monster ··········60
	The MTHFR Gene Mutation (No, it's not short for a bad word.)···············61
Chapter 5	The Playground Bully inside Your Nervous System ·······65
	The Autonomic Nervous System ············66

Pedal to the Medal: The One Thing Every Single CRPS Patient's Nervous System Has in Common · · · · · · · · · · · · ·68
The Sympathetic Nervous System: "Fight or Flight" · · · · · · 69
The Parasympathetic Nervous System: "Rest and digest" Or "Feed and breed" · 70
The Vagus Nerve: Your Severed Lifeline · · · · · · · · · · · · · · · 71
Your Achy Breaky Heart · 72
Just Breathe: How the Vagus Nerve Affects Your Lungs · · · 73
Gut Feelings Are Actually Real: How the Vagus Nerve Connects with Your Emotions· 74
Jeepers Creepers: How Unhealthy Gut Bacteria Control You and Your Habits · 75
Leaky Gut and Allergies · 76
When Eating Becomes Torture: The Vagus Nerve and Your Digestive System · 77
Sleep, a Distant Memory · 78
Avoid Blue Lights (and we aren't talking about the police.)· · · 79
Exhaustion · 80
Signs of Adrenal Fatigue · 81
How to Get Tested for Adrenal Fatigue at Home · · · · · · · · 82
Another Test I Recommend: Saliva Testing · · · · · · · · · · · · · 83
Underactive Thyroid (or why looking at a cookie makes you gain two pounds)· 84
Remember: The nervous system of a CRPS sufferer is often stuck in sympathetic overdrive.· · · · · · · · · · · · · · · · · · · 85
Signs of a thyroid that isn't working · · · · · · · · · · · · · · · · · · 85
How to Get Tested for a Sluggish Thyroid? Have Both T3 and T4 Tested · 86
TSH: The Old Guard's Way· 86
Thyroid Antibody Test · 87
Reverse T3 (aka triiodothyronine)· 87
The Temperature Test· 88
Is Your Thyroid Slow Or Your Adrenals Low? (or Both?) · · · 88

Chapter 6 Slow Fire Burn: The Role of Inflammation in CRPS · · · · · · · · ·91
           All the Other Players Responsible for Inflammation · · · · · · · ·93
                Histamine ·93
                Neutrophils ·93
                T-cells ·93
                Macrophages ·94
                Cytokines ·94
                Free Radicals ·95
                Nitric Oxide (NO) ·96
           The Role of the Vagus Nerve ·97
           The Atlas and the Vagus Nerve ·97
           Vagal Tone ·98
           Vagus Nerve and CRPS ·98
           How Chronic Inflammation Causes Pain in CRPS · · · · · · · ·100
           Sympathetic Sprouting ·101
           Sympathetically Maintained Pain (SMP) · · · · · · · · · · · · · ·101
           Painful Triggers ·102
           The Dreadful Spread ·102
           Other Possible Inflammation Triggers or Contributors
           Toxicity ·103
           What Are Toxins? ·104
           Heavy Metals ·105
           Heavy Metal/Candida Link ·108
           The Danger in Your Mouth ·109
           Amalgam Fillings ·110
           Root Canals ·111
           CRPS Patients Beware! ·113
           How to Test for Cellular Inflammation? · · · · · · · · · · · · · ·113
           Let's Recap ·114
Chapter 7 Pain, Your Dark Passenger ·115
           Toxic Lesions of the Disc(s) in the Neck · · · · · · · · · · · · · · · · ·115
           Substance P (Think P for Pain) ·117
           Central Sensitization ·117

Two Pillars of the Same Bridge: How Tailbone or Low Back injuries May Affect the Neck · · · · · · · · · · · · · · · · · 118
Cervical Spine Stenosis: Does It Make You Vulnerable to Damage? · 120
Congenital Stenosis of the Cervical Spinal Canal · · · · · · · 121
Degenerative Stenosis of the Cervical Spinal Canal · · · · · 121
How Do I Know if My Neck Is the Problem? · · · · · · · · · · · · 122
Central Pain · 122
Weather Changes · 123
How Can I Be Tested? · 124
Cervical X-Rays · 124
MRI · 125
Functional MRI · 126
Myelogram · 126
Physical and Neurological Exams · 126

Chapter 8 As If CRPS Is Not Enough: Coexistent Conditions Adding to Your Misery · 128
Allergies · 129
Chronic Fatigue Syndrome · 130
Digestive Disorders · 130
The Basic Steps Necessary to Heal the Digestive System · 132
Fibromyalgia · 132
Rheumatoid Arthritis (RA) · 133
Post-Traumatic Stress Disorder (PTSD) · · · · · · · · · · · · · · · 133
Multiple Sclerosis (MS) · 134
Lyme Disease · 135
Treatment Steps for Lyme Disease · · · · · · · · · · · · · · · · · · 136
Interstitial Cystitis (CS) · 137
Trigeminal Neuralgia · 138
Restless Leg Syndrome · 138
Ehlers-Danlos Syndrome · 139
Postural Orthostatic Tachycardia Syndrome (POTS) · · · · · 139
Vulvodynia · 140

	Weird Chest Pain · 140
	Changes to Your Brain · 140
Chapter 9	The Old Way: Current Diagnosis and Treatment Methods of CRPS · 142
	The Most Confusing Part: Obtaining a Diagnosis · · · · · · · 142
	The Three-Phase Bone Scan · 143
	X-Rays · 144
	CRPS and Bone Loss · 144
	Thermogram · 144
	Neurologic Tests · 145
	Physical Exam · 146
	Navigating the Confusing Maze of Treatments · · · · · · · · · 147
	Pain Medication · 148
	Opioids · 149
	Lyrica · 149
	Cymbalta · 150
	Low Dose Naltrexone (LDN) · 150
	All the others · 151
	Calmare Therapy · 152
	Ketamine · 153
	Spinal-Cord Stimulators · 155
	Pain (Drug) Pumps · 156
	Sympathectomy · 157
	Transcranial Magnetic Stimulation · · · · · · · · · · · · · · · · 158
	Neridronate · 158
	Hyperbaric Chambers · 160
	Marijuana · 161
Chapter 10	A New Way: Healing the Central Nervous System · · · · · · 163
	What Makes Our Treatment Different? · · · · · · · · · · · · · · 164
	The Secret Sauce · 165
	Exposing The Makings of a Monster: Testing · · · · · · · · · · 167
	Surface Electromyography Exam (SEMG) · · · · · · · · · · · · 168
	Heart Rate Variability (HRV) Exam · · · · · · · · · · · · · · · · 168

Full-Spine X-Rays	169
Meta-Oxy inflammation test	169
Heavy-Metal Urine Test	170
The Four-Punch System	170
First Punch: Waking Up the Vagus Nerve	171
Second Punch: Frequency Specific Microcurrent (FSM)	173
Third Punch: Rehabilitating the Nervous System	175
Fourth Punch: Increasing Circulation	177
Other Things	178
Chapter 11 Give Your Body a Fighting Chance: Your Diet	179
What Is Your pH? Acid versus Alkaline	181
It's All about Omega-3/Omega-6s	183
Your Cells on Fire: The Role of Cellular Inflammation	184
Animals Are What They Eat: Try to Keep Your Animal Products Natural	185
Watch Those Carbs	185
Avoid Carbs And Bring On The Fat: Ketogenic Diet	187
Bottoms Up	187
It Takes More Than One Apple a Day	188
Fats Don't Make You Fat.	190
Saturated Fats	191
Unsaturated Fats	191
Hydrogenated and Partially Hydrogenated Fats	191
Trans-fatty Acids	192
Allergies and Other Irritating Foods	192
The Exception to the 80/20 rule: The No-No List	194
Chapter 12 The Supplement Maze: Where to Begin?	196
Whole-food Multivitamin	199
Vitamin D3	201
Vitamin K2 (Your Calcium Taxi)	202
Glutathione	203
N-Acetyl Cysteine	204
Alpha Lipoic Acid	205

  Fish Oil · 205
  Freeze-Dried Aloe Vera · 206
  Pomegranate Juice · 207
  Adrenal Support · 208
  Methylfolate (5-methyltetrahydrofolate [5-MTHF]) · · · · · · 208
  Magnesium (Your "Stress Mineral") · · · · · · · · · · · · · · · · 209
  Selenium · 209
  Ubiquinol (or Coenzyme Q10) · 210
  Acetyl-L-Carnitine · 211
  D-Ribose · 212
  Malic Acid · 212
  Curcumin · 212
  Zinc · 213
Chapter 13 Tales from the War Front: Real Patient Stories · · · · · · · · 214
  Carlos Jasso's Story · 214
  David Smith's Story · 217
  How It All Started · 217
  The Meds · 218
  The Financial Blessings and Challenges · · · · · · · · · · · · · 218
  The Mental and Emotional fallout · · · · · · · · · · · · · · · · · 219
  Hope Lost · 219
  Never, Ever, Give Up! · 220
  The Consult · 221
  An Unexpected Benefit · 222
  Results · 222
  Brenda's Story · 223
  Barbara Wall's story · 226
Chapter 14 Don't. You. Ever. Stop. Fighting. · · · · · · · · · · · · · · · · · · · 230
  What You Focus on Expands · 233
  Repeat after Me: Doctors Work for You, Not the Other
  Way Around · 234
  What Does Remission Look Like? · · · · · · · · · · · · · · · · · 235
  Characteristics of Healing · 236

Parting Words of Wisdom · 240

Acknowledgements · 247
Other Book By This Author · 249
References · 251

Foreword

If you are reading this, you or someone you love is suffering from RSD/CRPS. My heart goes out to you. If you are the sufferer, no one can comprehend your suffering unless he or she shares your diagnosis. Your pain is your dark passenger, often invisible, yet a hell that is all too real. If you care about someone who suffers from RSD/CRPS, you bear witness to his or her pain. You stand by helplessly, watching your loved one being burned alive by this monster. It is my most sincere wish that this book will bring you comfort of even the smallest measure.

Whether you or a family member suffers from RSD/CRPS, I sincerely hope that this book will give you some of the answers you have long been searching for about your own condition or perhaps provide you with tools to help better understand the pain and symptoms of someone you care about. As a friend or family member of someone with RSD/CRPS, there is no greater gift you can give him or her than the gift of compassion and caring. Knowledge leads to sympathy and better understanding and being able to support them better.

As a person who suffers from RSD/CRPS, you have probably found that much in your life is no longer under your control. You have most likely been to a lot of doctors over time, many of whom may not have understood your condition. In addition, mind-numbing daily pain may have robbed you of many of the pleasurable things you once enjoyed. You may sometimes feel as if you are the only person in the world suffering from this horrible condition, something that very few doctors truly understand.

Overall, it is my hope for you to gain a sense of control over this condition. I want you to walk away from this book empowered. In order to do this, I will lead you through what I believe causes RSD/CRPS, its history, and its inner workings. In addition, I will provide you with practical steps that will allow you to beat this beast down. I hope to provide you with brand-new, practical information.

Before we delve in, I first want to discuss some of the unique characteristics surrounding RSD/CRPS. These make it one of the most difficult, challenging, and complicated conditions to work with and to suffer from.

- Very few people understand daily chronic pain, not to mention RSD/CRPS. RSD/CRPS is like an uninvited bully quietly taking possession of your body. It rarely shows its face to the world as it tears you apart from the inside. When people first find out, they usually try. However, as the weeks, months, and years go by, they run out of things to tell you in order to comfort you. As a result, they start pretending that you are OK, and they want you to do the same.
- In general, few doctors truly understand RSD/CRPS. Before patients are first diagnosed, they must navigate an endless maze of specialists, often painful tests, and misdiagnoses. If you are lucky enough to have been diagnosed relatively quickly, your options are few and limited. A lot of medical professionals have never heard of RSD/CRPS. Even if they have heard about it, they still misunderstand it (e.g., thinking that RSD/CRPS can't spread).
- Most doctors and other medical professionals are very skeptical of daily chronic pain. This is not really their fault, as so many people abuse the system to get high. It is hard when you are in real pain, however, and stigmatized on top of it. Think of it as earning your black belt in RSD/CRPS. You most probably will be suspected of being a lying, drug-seeking junkie at least once.
- Most doctors "treat" RSD/CRPS by throwing drugs at it. These drugs or medications (at best) will (somewhat) cover up your symptoms. In the case of RSD/CRPS, it's usually far from the perfect solution,

although it may provide some relief. I have yet to meet any patient who told me that he or she, or someone he or she knew, was "cured" by any drug. Furthermore, every drug has side effects. That being said, I understand that drugs may feel like your only saving grace right now and that for some of you they are lifesavers. They may make the difference between you getting out of bed in the morning and (kind of) living a halfway normal life, or not.

- Most recognized RSD/CRPS treatments available on the market today (or soon to be available) involve the numbing, scrambling, or interruption of pain signals.
- People who suffer from RSD/CRPS often feel all alone and even ashamed. They feel that some people may think that they just want sympathy or that it's all in their heads. Since RSD/CRPS is invisible in most cases, patients suffering from it still feel as if they have to prove that they really are suffering. Even if people do believe you, it's not as if they can ever fully comprehend your daily unrelenting level of suffering. Childbirth? Yeah, that ends, and you get to hold your brand-new baby in the end. There is no pot of gold at the end of this rainbow. Migraines? They are little puppies compared to the rabid beast that is RSD/CRPS. In addition, most people have never heard of this condition outside of the RSD/CRPS community. Let's be honest—as far as diseases and conditions go, RSD/CRPS is not a trendy or popular one.
- Often, your family and friends don't understand. It doesn't matter how much they love you or how supportive they are. At the end of the day, living with RSD/CRPS is like being in a prison all alone. You can see through the bars, but you can't escape. No one can climb inside your body and feel the pain you suffer every day or understand how life-robbing it is.
- All RSD/CRPS patients (understandably) hope, pray, or wish for a cure. This magical cure is like a fabled unicorn…much discussed but elusive if you actually want to touch it. This cure is expected to be presented in the form of a surgery, infusion, or drug.

- RSD/CRPS patients themselves often do not fully understand all the symptoms that may be associated with their condition. Digestive issues anyone? Are you a walking weather detector? Do you cringe when a baby cries at the grocery store? Internal thermometer all screwy? Trouble swallowing? Digestive issues? Does the pain from something as simple as taking a shower (instead of being warm and relaxing) put you over the edge each time? Do you dread just washing your hair? Yes. Chances are this laundry list of symptoms from hell is most often all connected.
- Most people suffering from RSD/CRPS have considered (at least once) to end it all. Patients are ashamed of this and often this is not openly discussed. However, know that you are probably not alone. I will discuss this more in chapter 3.
- Patients suffering from RSD/CRPS experience intense guilt. There are many reasons for this. They may feel like a burden or worry about their family members' concern for them. They feel guilty for not being fun, for interfering with family activities, for being a financial drain, for not wanting to have sex, for being in bed, for always being tired, and for not being able to dance. The list of guilt-inducing reasons is as long as their arm.

It isn't fair. I know. If you were diagnosed with, let's say, breast cancer, you wouldn't have to go around educating the world about your condition and assuring them that yes, breast cancer *is* real. You wouldn't feel ashamed. You wouldn't make excuses. Your doctor would understand your symptoms. You wouldn't be so alone. I understand, I really do. However, today, you have reached a fork in the road. You chose this book. That shows me that at the very least, you have the desire to still learn. At most, I hope that this book is the beginning of you getting your life back again. At the very least, I hope it brings you understanding about your condition. There is an old Chinese proverb that says every journey begins with a single step. I look forward to this journey with you.

My Story

Great opportunities to help others seldom come.

—SALLY KOCH

You never know how far reaching something you may think, say or do today will affect the lives of millions tomorrow.

—B. J. PALMER

I am not sure what your spiritual beliefs are. One of mine, which I hold sacred, is this—each of us was put upon this earth with a very specific mission and purpose. I believe that we are *meant* to make a difference and to make the world a better place, and that we are meant to live our passion and touch others' lives with it. This is the story of how I found mine.

I was born and raised in Johannesburg, South Africa. I was blessed to have been born to a chiropractic dad and a mother who, once she was exposed to a natural health style, really embraced the philosophy of healthy organic eating and preventative care. Except for emergencies, I was raised with the philosophy that the body is a self-healing, self-regulating organism and can usually heal without medications or shots. The only time we kids would see the doctor was when my brothers needed stitches—which, given that they were typical boys, was quite often.

My family's love of chiropractic is deeply rooted. When my father was seven years old, my grandparents were told not to expect him to survive into adulthood, due to very severe allergies. At the time, my grandfather, a very hard-working cattle rancher, had been saved from back surgery by a local chiropractor, after his brothers literally carried him out of the hospital into the chiropractor's office. My grandparents wondered if chiropractic care could perhaps help my dad, and they took him along the next time my grandfather had an appointment. Sixty-seven years later, my dad is still very much alive and allergy-free.

Because my dad's life was saved by chiropractic, he felt passionately "called" into that profession. When he was twenty-one, he left South Africa to attend Palmer College of Chiropractic in Davenport, Iowa. He graduated at the age of twenty-four, at which time he went back to South Africa and went on to become extremely successful.

When I was three years old, I climbed onto my dad's big chair behind his desk and announced to my parents that I would be a chiropractor one day. From that point on, I never considered another career. (As it turned out, I became a pretty good oil artist. People would urge me to study art and sell my paintings. I resisted, resolute in my career of choice.) I started chiropractic school in Johannesburg in 1994.

When my family immigrated to the United States in 1994, my dad left behind a thriving practice and many beloved patients. Part of the reason we moved here was because my dad always said that, while he was helping about eight out of every ten patients, he finally found himself consumed by the two out of ten whom he *couldn't* help. Eventually, helping those patients with more complicated conditions became an obsession for him, which I in turn inherited. He felt that moving to the United States would afford him with more opportunities to stay on the cutting edge of treatments, techniques, research, and training.

Leaving school, I joined my dad in practice in northwest Arkansas, close to where Walmart is headquartered. It is a lovely, thriving area, and yet I considered it to be only a pit stop while I figured out where in the United States I wanted to settle. After all, I have always lived around big cities. As it turned out, I never left. Later, my younger sister joined us in practice.

From the beginning, practicing as a chiropractor was disappointing to me. I quickly became burned out. Teaching a natural, preventative approach to health (as is the chiropractic school of thought), rather than practicing disease care, is incredibly frustrating. My patients were bombarded by pharmaceutical companies using relentless marketing tools. An age-old model for this is used very successfully: create fear, and then offer a solution (e.g., create fear of the flu, and then offer this season's flu vaccine). In addition, most people had little interest in eating a healthier diet or exercising or investing in preventative health tools such as vitamins and chiropractic.

Another frustrating thing was the type of patients I was treating. While most of them were great people, I found myself plodding along in mind-numbing symptom mud, consisting of back pain, neck pain, herniated discs, sciatica, and the occasional headache. How was I going to save lives? How was I going to pull people out of desperation when most people weren't even convinced that they needed chiropractic in order to be healthier? My soul longed for more. I needed some purpose. I needed something bigger than myself.

For eight years I practiced like this. I was deeply unhappy and trying to deny it. All around me, I heard chiropractic and spiritual gurus talk about "finding your purpose" and "living passionately." How I wanted that... my soul cried out for it, but in practice, that was not my reality. I went as far as writing out a mission statement and hanging it above my desk. It described in detail how passionate I was about my work and how I was helping people. The only problem was that I could not lie to myself. Deep down, I knew I was a fraud.

You see, chiropractors typically walk a difficult path. Practicing in a world driven by people seeking immediate relief and thinking in an allopathic way can be very tough. When you choose to become an alternative health-care provider, you are going against the grain, trying to do your own small part to make people healthier from the inside out, not the outside in. You are like a soldier, fighting for people to begin to understand that their bodies can heal and repair themselves and must be kept in good order *before* they get sick. Chiropractors are sometimes called "oh" doctors, as in, "What kind of doctor are you? Oh…" Despite the widespread myth that the chiropractor's education is somehow inferior to that of a medical doctor (not true!) or that they are "bone poppers" (or maybe because of it), chiropractors tend to be very passionate about what they do. Most chiropractors can tell you the second they were "called" into their profession. I just seemed to be born into it. I began to wonder if perhaps I chose my profession only in an effort to please my dad.

My doubts grew stronger as I became more miserable. I had a hole in my life, and it was called Lacking Passion. Completely burned out, I started to think of other ways I could make a living. Then, about five years ago, I received an e-mail about a supposedly amazing technique, getting amazing results with, among other conditions, fibromyalgia as well as RSD/CRPS. Very skeptically, I attended a webinar and listened in disbelief to the results these doctors were reporting. A week later, I attended the seminar. While at that seminar, something woke up inside of me. It was passion. Excitement. Understanding. A passion to help the hopeless.

When I came home, I was seeing absolute astounding results treating the neurologic symptoms of fibromyalgia. Encouraged and curious, I tracked down my first local RSD/CRPS patient, Jenni. I invited her to my office to let me try this technique on her and she agreed. I was convinced that I was going to change her life. She came in, I explained the procedure, and we got to work. Drum roll. I expected so much, and her pain… did not change at all. I was devastated. She was resigned; after all, she didn't expect much. I kept doggedly trying for a week. Finally, after developing a severe migraine (not uncommon for her) she gave up. Luckily, our story didn't end there. Jenni taught me so much about tenacity, about educating myself, about not ever giving up. Boy, was I green (but more about her later).

Luckily, I didn't give up treating RSD/CRPS after Jenni. My very next patient was Carlos, a full-body RSD/CRPS patient. My treatment of him proved to be a raging success right off the bat, and I felt as if I have finally discovered my true passion. I wanted to help the hopeless, and no chronic pain condition was more hopeless than RSD/CRPS. In my experience, no doctor can truly "see" the horror of RSD/CRPS without becoming completely obsessed with helping those who suffer from it. I was no different. This was the condition that I have been waiting for. I set out to become the best at what I did, to find the giants treating the suspected *cause* of neurologic dysfunction resulting in RSD/CRPS rather than the symptoms. I traveled. I studied. I became obsessed and I was actually helping people. A lot.

In 2012, I realized that I had to reach more patients. I wrote my first book *Taming the Beast: A Guide to Conquering Fibromyalgia*, and I reached tons of people. Our Facebook group grew to ten thousand plus members. Word of mouth increased. Slowly but surely, the RSD/CRPS patients also started coming and we kept seeing miracles. I kept refining my treatment into a whole-body approach, while always holding fast to my philosophy—don't treat or suppress the pain, treat the *cause* of neurologic dysfunction. It's been five years since placing my hands on my first RSD/CRPS patient. My life since has been completely transformed.

Many of my patients have told me that had it not been for my treatment, they would have committed suicide. How privileged am I, that I get the chance to change and save lives? It's like throwing a rock in the pond, where the ripple effect goes on beyond your understanding. When people get their lives back, the effects of it are far-reaching. *Everyone* around them is affected. Patients may return to work, or to their hobbies. They can be good friends, grandparents, husbands, wives, brothers and sisters again. Patients can return to fully *living* once more. I make it my life's mission to keep my skills and education current and cutting-edge, often ahead of what the masses know. I am constantly learning. My other job, which I charged myself with, is delivering that knowledge to those who need it. I want to make a difference.

I am incredibly blessed. I have found my passion: helping those in chronic, debilitating pain. Helping those with RSD/CRPS is a burning flame of passion in my heart. Every day, my patients tell me that I should reach more people. At least once a month, someone asks me "if this is so great, and so many people are suffering from RSD/CRPS, why do so few know about you?" They are right. People should know about my work. I have knowledge in my heart and head that must be shared with you. I found my passion, and I can never go back to a life without it. In addition, I know that I cannot keep this miracle that I have discovered to myself, nor share it with just a lucky few. Because of this knowledge, this passion, and this *knowing*, I sat down this morning and started writing this book. Hopefully, because of it, I will get to touch your life too.

—Dr. Katinka

1

The Basics: Understanding the Nature of the Monster

It is such a mysterious place, the land of tears....

—Antoine de Saint-Exupéry, *The Little Prince*

If hell were a clinical condition, it might look something like reflex sympathetic dystrophy or RSD.

—Tom Haederle, Johns Hopkins University

TRACING THE MONSTER'S FOOTPRINTS THROUGH HISTORY

It is my sincere belief that a patient has to understand his or her own condition from the ground up, inside out. Even though RSD/CRPS is an unwelcome houseguest, it would still behoove you to know what exactly you are unwillingly coexisting with. In my experience, patients who eventually recover work hard to understand their own condition. Therefore, we will dissect this monster and attempt to understand its beginnings.

The first descriptions of RSD/CRPS were documented by a young US Army contract physician, Silas Weir Mitchell, MD. Dr. Mitchell treated soldiers suffering from gunshot wounds. In his book *Gunshot wounds, and Other Injuries*, he documents pain that persisted long after the bullets were removed and the wounds appeared to be healed. He described that this pain was characteristic in that it was "burning" in nature. Because of this, his friend Robley Dunglison coined the term "Causalgia" (Greek for burning pain). Dr. Mitchell speculated that CRPS was caused by nerve injury suffered after trauma.

> *Under such torments, the temper changes, the most amiable grow irritable, the soldier becomes a coward, and the strongest man is scarcely less nervous than the most hysterical girl.*
>
> —Silas Weir Mitchell, MD

Dr. Mitchell (much like doctors today) was perplexed by the phenomenon of ongoing, relentless sympathetic pain. He painstakingly recorded case after case of causalgia in his 1872 book, *Injuries of Nerves and Their Consequences*. Mitchell noted that the pain varied in location from patient to patient, but that "its favorite site is the foot or hand." He also noted that many reported, together with the pain, a peculiar glossiness of the skin, and that most patients avoided exposing the painful area to dry air at all costs. Most of his patients were strong, healthy men before they were injured, who found their lives forever changed after.

> *As the pain increase, the general sympathy becomes more marked. The temper changes and grows irritable, the face becomes anxious, and has a look of weariness and suffering. The sleep is restless, and the constitutional condition, reacting on the wounded limb, exasperates the hyperaesthetic state, so that the rattling of a newspaper, a breath of air…the vibrations caused by a military band, or the shock of feet in walking, gives rise to increased pain. At last…the patient walks carefully, carries the limb with the sound hand, is tremulous, nervous, and has all kinds of expedients for lessening his pain.*
>
> —Silas Weir Mitchell, MD

René Leriche, MD, was a military surgeon also, who treated many WWI soldiers exhibiting the same type of symptoms after the initial trauma that Dr. Mitchell noted. Dr. Leriche initially treated this pain with sympathectomies (an irreversible procedure in which at least one sympathetic ganglion is permanently removed). Later, he treated the condition with "novocain infiltrations." As with many physicians who specialize in treating RSD/CRPS, he was tormented by his patients' suffering, and consequently wrote a book titled *La Chirurgie de la Douleur* (Surgery of Pain).

Another military doctor, William K. Livingston, MD treated peripheral nerve injuries during WWII. He noted "the vicious circle of pain as similar with vasoconstriction and atrophy." He also noted that the contralateral limb would often become symptomatic.

All through history, and all across the world, descriptions or the study of RSD/CRPS and its treatment can be found. In 1890, a French neurologist by the name of Jean-Martin Charcot (considered by some to be the founder of modern neurology) noted that the disease was accompanied by "nonpitting edema, changes in color, changes in skin temperature, tenderness of the skin and pain." Although these were accurate and useful observations, he was of the opinion that this condition was caused by self-suggestion, which is just another way of saying it's all in your head. Note a pattern? In 1900, Dr. Sudeck, a German surgeon, discovered that patients often suffered from osteoporosis, starting in the small bones of the hands and feet and eventually spreading. These changes could be seen on x-ray. Sudeck theorized that RSD/CRPS could be caused by an acute inflammatory response after an injury.

In 1947, Dr. Steinbrocker renamed the disease as "shoulder-hand syndrome," and treated the disease with oral corticosteroids. In 1974, Dr. Hannington-Kiff pioneered the use of IV blocks of the sympathetic nervous system, still in use today. In the 1990s, Dr. R. J. A. Goris, a Dutch surgeon and scientist, pioneered modern study of CRPS-I, the subtype thought at the time to not exhibit any nerve injury. In addition to phenotyping,[1] he also identified the first evidence of nerve injuries.[2] In 1993, a special consensus workshop held in Florida provided the now widely accepted "Complex Regional Pain Syndrome."

Today, numerous new treatments are available with varying degrees of success. As I write this, newer treatments yet are being investigated. The one thing most of these treatments share is that they all interrupt, scramble, or numb the pain. Other treatments involve physical therapy, psychological support, and neuromodulation. Results are usually unsatisfactory, especially if begun late in the game. Later on in this book, we will go on to discuss most of the most well-known treatments.

As for suffering from RSD/CRPS today, one may count a few blessings after all. Today, RSD/CRPS has a color and a ribbon (it is orange). There are numerous organizations, books, support groups, and resources available. Famous people have stepped forward to give this condition a face (e.g., US ski champion Jill Boothe and singer and TV personality Paula Abdul).

The Internet united millions of RSD/CRPS sufferers worldwide. It served to mobilize, connect, and promote knowledge of the condition. It is easy to imagine a poor, desperate soul futilely suffering in the middle ages, or ancient Egypt. Back then, these people must have felt all alone and misunderstood. There were no treatments, no support groups, and no help to be had. Even in today's age, there are places in this world where others suffering the same hell you suffer are not so lucky. A poor villager in an underdeveloped country in Africa is lucky to get even the most basic life-saving medical care, not to mention a doctor who can diagnose, understand or treat CRPS. Whenever I go to Mexico on vacation, one of my favorite countries, I often wonder how many people with no resources within a five-hundred-mile radius of my beautiful hotel are suffering silent lives of untold pain. I imagine these people to be cut off from any understanding, progress, or support from the worldwide CRPS community. It simply breaks my heart.

If you were in a position to somehow hear or read about this book, for example, chances are that you are already blessed, compared to other CRPS patients. The most important weapon you have today is the ability to have access to the Internet and with a few keystrokes, reach millions of people suffering from the same thing you suffer from. Word of mouth is an amazing tool. All you need is knowledge, the refusal to give up, and a perpetually open mind.

DECONSTRUCTING THE MONSTER

Through history, many different names have been associated with CRPS. Some of these include reflex sympathetic dystrophy, causalgia, peripheral trophoneurosis, minor traumatic dystrophy, atrophie de Sudeck, and algodystrophy, to name a few. For the purpose of simplicity, we will refer to RSD/CRPS as simply CRPS henceforth. Many more women seem to suffer from CRPS than men (about 75 percent more). CRPS has been diagnosed in very young children (so much for it being a "manufactured" condition) and usually peaks around midlife. It is a chronic disease that often worsens over time. Alarmingly, 35 percent of sufferers eventually report symptoms throughout the body. The disease may remain localized, spread slowly over years, or progress rapidly like a wildfire out of control.

CRPS is associated with imbalance and malfunction of the autonomic nervous system resulting in disability, impairment, chronic pain, and functional loss. The International Association for the Study of Pain has proposed dividing CRPS into two types.

- Type I, formerly known as Sudeck's atrophy or reflex sympathetic dystrophy (RSD) does not exhibit demonstrable nerve lesions. The vast majority of people suffering from CRPS have this type.
- Type II, formerly known as causalgia, has obvious nerve damage present. As a rule, type II is considered the more painful of the two types with an unenviable 47/50 score on the McGill pain scale.

While CRPS was considered in the past to have three stages, it is now believed that patients with CRPS do not necessarily progress through these stages, or progress sequentially.

- Stage 1 is characterized by intense, burning pain at the site of injury. Muscle spasms, joint stiffness, swelling, restricted mobility, vasospasms, rapid nail and hair growth, decrease in temperature, and decreased range of motion have all been reported. This has also been called "wet CRPS" as some patients may experience increased sweating. For a few lucky patients, this stage may last for a few weeks and then resolve on its own. For the unlucky majority, it progresses.
- Stage 2 is characterized by even more intense pain, described by some as similar to the sensation of burning alive or being burned with a blowtorch. Hair growth is inhibited; swelling spreads; osteoporosis becomes severe; nails may crack, pit, grooved or have spots on them; joints tend to thicken, and the muscles will atrophy or shrink, causing the affected limb to appear thinner than the other.

- Stage 3 is characterized by permanent changes in the skin and bones, while the pain becomes even more intense and now may involve the entire limb. Flexor tendon contractions may be present causing the limb or appendage to contract (much like a claw). The symptoms may spread to any other body part, for example the optic nerves or the digestive system.

THE ROLL OF THE GENETIC DICE: IS CRPS HEREDITARY?

While a familial occurrence in the development of CRPS has not been extensively studied, at least one study[3] suggests that such a link is present. Through my years of treating this disease, I have treated or been in touch with multiple families struck more than once by CRPS. It is interesting to me that in math, angles are said to coincide if they are congruent, meaning; their corresponding angles, sides and occupied areas are *exactly* equal. The word "coincidence" therefore often hints at something that is exactly the opposite of "accidently" or "by random chance."

Further, it has been theorized that between five and eight million people worldwide suffer from CRPS. Considering all the people who do not have access to superior medical care, the relative failure of such superior medical care when it comes to the accurate and timely diagnoses of CRPS, and all the people in underdeveloped and underprivileged areas who may never have been to a doctor, clinic or hospital, never mind diagnosed, it stands to reason that that number may be much, much higher. Despite that fact, if you consider that the world population has now exceeded seven billion people, it seems like too much of a coincidence that CRPS will strike the same family more than once.

Donald A. Rhodes DPM, who designed one of the treatment systems I use in my clinic, called the Vecttor, introduced me to the following information:

The autonomic nervous system and various neuropeptides control the circulation in the body. Neuropeptides are small protein-like molecules used by nerve cells in order to communicate with each other. VIP (vasoactive intestinal polypeptide) is a chemical found in the human body that increases the blood flow to the intestines. The flow of blood to the skin, nerves, bones and small muscles is increased by yet another peptide, called CGRP (calcitonin gene-related peptide). As they say, what goes up, must come down, and as the body always seeks balance, this increased blood flow is, in turn, decreased by substance P, elsewhere referred to in this book. Substance P causes specialized cells called mast cells to release an enzyme that destroys CGRP. In healthy individuals, there is a balance between norepinephrine and substance P, which decrease blood flow to various tissues and organs, while CGRP and VIP increase the blood flow in return. Norepinephrine is an organic chemical that functions in the human brain and body as a hormone and a neurotransmitter, or messenger. It is released by the central nervous system. Norepinephrine is destroyed on a system-wide basis by catecholO-methyltransferase (COMT).

The amount of COMT produced by the body is determined by an individual's genetic makeup. Dr. Jan Zubieta performed groundbreaking research on the action of COMT genes. A variation in genetics determines how individuals respond to pain. It also determines how long norepinephrine produced by the sympathetic nervous system last in the body. When he studied those complaining of severe pain, he found that most of these individuals fall within a 25 percent segment of the population that have a specific combination of COMT genes. In these patients, norepinephrine remains active in the body for much longer periods of time.

It has been found that the bulk of fibromyalgia and CRPS patients (as well as other forms of chronic pain) are patients with abnormally low levels of COMT. This increased duration of the action of norepinephrine causes decreased circulation in the skin, GI tract, nerves, bones, and small muscles. In turn, this causes ischemia. Ischemia is decreased circulation causing decreased available oxygen in tissues. Many of these diseases affect women more than men, as men tend to have higher blood pressure as a rule of thumb. In addition, men generally have more muscle mass and therefore more myoglobin, which "holds" oxygen in the muscles. These patients may also suffer from related conditions such as Raynaud's phenomenon, a condition marked by cold hands and feet, as well as POTS, as mentioned in chapter 8.

In addition, there is a fairly high rate of comorbidity present between CRPS and fibromyalgia, as these two conditions often share similar central nervous system dysfunction as described in chapter 6. The hereditary nature of fibromyalgia has been demonstrated more clearly than in the case of CRPS. Below are some examples of research that backs this genetic hypothesis up.

- The Swedish Twin Registry reports that there is up to a 15 percent higher chance of one twin developing fibromyalgia if the other twin suffers from it.
- Studies suggested that fibromyalgia segregates within families in an autosomal dominant mode of inheritance. One of them[4] showed female preponderance and, in addition, postulated the existence of a latent or precursor stage of the disease characterized by abnormal muscle tension.
- Another study[5] was based on data retrieved from questionnaires regarding fibromyalgia symptoms in family members of index patients. According to this study, about two-thirds of the study population reported family clustering.

So what does all this research mean? If you have family members with fibromyalgia or CRPS, there may be a higher chance of you developing the condition(s), or your children one day suffering from the same pain. However, all is not hopeless. The noted scientist Bruce Lipton, PhD, is one of many scientists today proving that we are, in fact, not victims of our genetic material. Dr. Lipton is a well-respected cellular biologist who has done extensive research at Stanford University on the mechanics of genetics and cellular biology.

Most of us were taught that the genetic blueprint we inherited from our parents predetermines our bodies, our personalities, our talents, and even our health. But in the last two decades, Dr. Lipton and other cellular biologists have discovered that, while our genes do not change, the way they are *expressed* may be very much within our control. In layman's terms, this means that even though we may have a higher risk of developing certain conditions or diseases because of our biology, we have a lot of power to *minimize* those risks.

This is good news! Since Dr. Lipton first observed two cells with exactly the same genetic code, in two different petri dishes (different environments), behaving in very different ways, his work has become a foundation for scientific documentation of the mind-body connection. He explains that based on their genetic code, "cells can do a job that contributes to the growth of the organism, its maintenance, and keeping it healthy, or a cell can get into a position of a protection response. Cells need the brain to interpret the world and feed back to them what they should be doing to keep this whole system alive and floating."

According to Dr. Lipton, the true secret to life does not lie within your DNA, but rather within the mechanisms of your cell membrane. Each cell is surrounded by a membrane with receptors attached to it. Think of them as tiny cell phone towers receiving signals. These receptors pick up signals from their environment, which in turn control how the genes are read inside the cells. In other words, your cells can choose to read or ignore your genetic blueprint depending on the signals they receive from their environment. Simply put, this means that even potentially undesired cell behavior needs a very specific key to unlock it. This key is usually a physical, chemical, or emotional stress. The power to arm your body against this stress lies in your hands!

So, this means that having a "cancer program" or a "CRPS program" in your DNA does not mean you are destined to get cancer or develop CRPS. Isn't that good news? *You* control your environment to a large extent. You control your daily thoughts, your surroundings, your exercise habits, and your diet. You *do* have control over which genes are turned on and turned off. (For more on Dr. Lipton's work, go to www.brucelipton.com.)

If one or more of these conditions are present within your family, it will certainly be wise to be extra diligent after trauma (such as fractures) or surgery. In addition, it is so very important to eat a clean healthy diet, to supplement wisely, to learn how to respond to stress in a healthy manner, and to make absolutely sure that your central nervous system is in good working order and functioning at its optimal potential. Whiplash injuries must never be simply ignored. Please seek out the opinion of a good chiropractor to examine your central nervous system and spine as a precaution, as well as after any car accident, even if your X-ray doesn't show obvious trauma. If you contact us on Facebook or by phone, we will be happy to refer you or your family member to a local doctor.

2

The Bad and the Ugly: Mysterious Symptoms You May Not Associate with CRPS

Sometimes monsters are invisible, and sometimes demons attack you from the inside. Just because you cannot see the claws and the teeth does not mean they aren't ripping through me. Pain does not need to be seen to be felt. Telling me there is no problem won't solve the problem. This is not how miracles are born. This is not how sickness works.

—EMM ROY, THE FIRST STEP

In medical school, it's quite possible to get taught that you can diagnose everybody and treat everything. But then you get out in the real world and find that for most patients walking through your door, you have no idea what's causing their symptoms.

—BARRY MARSHALL

A good puzzle, it's a fair thing. Nobody is lying. It's very clear, and the problem depends just on you.

—ERNO RUBIK

The typical CRPS patient has been to many, many different doctors. They have navigated a maze of hospitals, clinics and specialists that most people cannot even begin to imagine the sheer volume of. They have been prodded, poked, stabbed (ill-advised for CRPS patients) and misdiagnosed many times. Chances are, they have been at least suspected (if not outright accused) of being pill-seeking junkies or malingering (a fancy medical word that basically means you are lying your butt off about your pain and symptoms.) The average CRPS patient will go misdiagnosed or undiagnosed for years before they are lucky enough to find out what is wrong with them. Many figure it out on their own with the help of the Internet, and have to then set out to prove it to their doctors. Who is responsible for your health? You are. Who cares most about your health? You do. It is *your* responsibility to make sense of your symptoms—to not only *understand* them, but to understand what is causing them.

Many doctors have never heard of CRPS and don't understand it. Even if patients are lucky enough to obtain an early diagnosis, finding successful treatment is as difficult as hunting a mythical unicorn down. Patients may spend thousands simply in co-pays and traveling cost only to be financially destroyed by the time they *do* find a promising treatment, usually not covered by insurance. It is frustrating, it is hard, and it is a rotten luck of the draw. However, one can sit down, or one can get back up. These are your choices. Keep fighting, be your own best advocate, or throw up your hands and hope it doesn't get worse and that someone will let you know on Facebook once they find a cure one day and that insurance will cover it.

I hope that doesn't sound harsh as I intend this to be a rallying speech, not a depressing one. In chapter 14, I will talk about the characteristics I have noticed all patients who recover from chronic pain share. For now though, we will talk about the first one. Patients have to understand their own symptoms and how they are connected. They have to know what they mean and how one problem links to another. It is my hope that this book will help you to navigate the symptom maze and leave you more savvy and educated than before. If a doctor wants to prescribe a medication to you for constipation, for example, you have to know why you are most likely constipated and if taking this medication is a smart move for you. You have to know if the medication has side effects and what they are. You can't ever trust anyone else to be a better steward of your body than you are. You can't expect others to guard your health better than you can.

In order to start unraveling your symptoms, we will look at the more common symptoms associated first, and then delve into the lesser known ones.

THE WELL-KNOWN SYMPTOMS

Over the years, diagnosing CRPS has changed quite a bit. These days, the Budapest criteria are often used to diagnose CRPS. These categories are most widely used and were developed by pain clinics to differentiate between CRPS and other neuropathic conditions (Harden et al., 2010). These look at four main categories of symptoms as shown below:

- Sensory abnormalities, such as an abnormal pain response to normal everyday sensory input. This includes directional pressure (such as being poked with a finger), light touch, circumferential pressure (such as putting on a tight sock), pain (being stabbed with a sharp object), cold, heat, exposure to humidity and vibration. Pain will also be perceived at a heightened intensity.
- Vasomotor abnormalities, which include differences in skin temperature greater than 1 degree Celsius, and a difference in skin color when comparing one part or limb of the body to the opposite part or limb.
- Sudomotor/edema, which include asymmetry in swelling and sweating.
- Motor/trophic, which is defined as decreased movement, muscle or nerve weakness, tremors, and changes in hair, skin or nails.

CRPS is identified by these symptoms in the following way:

- A: Ongoing pain that doesn't match the original injury in intensity or duration
- B: At least one symptom from two or more of the Budapest categories mentioned above
- C: At least one symptom from three or more of the four Budapest categories mentioned above
- D: A lack of alterative diagnosis

There are different tests that CRPS patients may have to endure in order to arrive at a final diagnosis of CRPS. These are discussed in detail in chapter 9. Next, I want to delve into the symptoms that often exist concurrently with CRPS, but that may not be commonly associated with it or may be treated as separate issues. It is important to note that these symptoms may be experienced in addition to the most common or obvious symptoms associated with CRPS. You may suffer from just a few, or if you are unlucky, from a long list of these.

Being a CRPS Expert Starts with You!
How to Make Sense of Your Body Gone Haywire

YOUR CRANIAL NERVES: THE FRONT DOOR TO YOUR NERVOUS SYSTEM

The cranial nerves are twelve pairs of nerves on the ventral (bottom) surface of the brain. These nerves control a lot of important things, and their purpose is mainly to connect you with the world around your body. Think of these nerves as your nervous system's front door to the world. These nerves allow you to hear, see, taste, and smell. Some of these nerves bring information from the sense organs to the brain. Some control muscles; others are connected to glands or internal organs such as the heart and lungs. One of the main functions of these nerves, in our caveman days and still today, is to perceive danger. We do this through our sensory nervous system. The cranial nerves in almost every CRPS patient show abnormalities. Here is how the malfunction of these important nerves may affect you:

- Loss of taste
- Speech disturbances, which can be so severe that it sounds as if you have suffered from a stroke (sometimes, you may have a hard time finding words or putting them in the right order)
- Balance loss
- A feeling of fullness in your ears
- Eye pain
- Burning in eyes
- Ever-changing eyesight and visual disturbances (if you are reading this book on an e-reader and had to change the font, this may be affecting you)
- Light sensitivity
- Blurred vision
- Feelings of disorientation, especially when going to a store like Costco or Sam's Club (these stores have large open spaces with no horizons, lots of visual stimulation, and the need for you to focus)
- Feelings of disorientation while in an elevator
- Fainting
- Light-headedness
- Nausea
- Carsickness or disorientation while riding in a car, especially when you look at strobe lights like the ones that emergency vehicles use
- Dizziness
- Ears ringing
- Ears buzzing
- Intolerance to loud sounds, such as a baby crying
- Hearing loss
- Inability to tolerate large crowds
- One-sided facial pain

- Pain in your teeth
- Jaw pain
- Difficulty swallowing
- Cystic acne
- Rashes
- Loss or thinning of lateral eyebrows
- Eyes appearing "buggy," like they are popping out
- Bags beneath your eyes
- Brown discoloration of patches of your skin (Melasma), commonly referred to as the "mask of pregnancy," when you are not pregnant

YOUR ACHY HEAD AND NECK

The cervical spine (neck) and any history of injuries to this area that you may have are so crucial that we will devote an entire chapter to them later. For now, let's just focus on your actual symptoms.

- Headaches
- Migraines
- One-sided headaches
- One-sided migraines
- Pain in back of head or base of skull
- Pain in either temple
- "Heavy" or "foggy" head
- Memory loss (One of my patients calls this CRPS Tourette's. Here is how she explained it: "Sometimes, things will pop into your head and then leave just as readily. Therefore, I have learned to spit it out the second I think of it. Sometimes my family will be discussing something completely unrelated to shopping, and I'd say "Apples! We need Apples!" Therefore, CRPS Tourette's.)
- Neck pain
- Pain when moving your neck

- Stiff neck
- Muscle spasm
- Neck "grinds" or "pops"
- Difficulty in moving the neck
- Nerves feel "pinched"
- Disc problems
- TMJ (temporomandibular joint) pain and problems
- Pain in the face (trigeminal neuralgia)
- Pain radiating into teeth
- Clenching your teeth at night
- Teeth grinding
- Pain that radiates into your teeth
- Pain when chewing food

BURDEN ON YOUR SHOULDERS

- Shoulder pain
- Rotator cuff problems
- Pain across your shoulders
- Tense or "hard" upper back and shoulder muscles, or what I refer to as "concrete shoulders" in my office
- Cannot lift either arm above the shoulder level
- Nerve pain or numbness in either (or both) shoulder(s)
- Tension in either (or both) shoulder(s)
- Pain in either (or both) arm(s)
- Forearm pain
- Finger pain
- Cold hands
- Inability to perform fine motor tasks (e.g., writing)
- Swelling in either (or both) hand(s)
- Pain in either (or both) wrist(s)
- Pain in either (or both) hand(s)

- Discoloration of fingers
- Fingernail changes
- Weak grip; for example, when opening bottles
- Dropping things a lot
- Tingling in any part of the upper extremities
- Burning in shoulders radiating from neck

MIDBACK AND CHEST

- Tender muscles in anterior chest
- Midback pain
- Pain when wearing a bra
- Pain between shoulder blades
- Midback spasms
- Pain when you get a massage
- Chest pain
- Pain in your breastbone
- Pain that feels like it's coming from your heart
- Shortness of breath
- Pain in your ribs (in the front or back)
- Difficulty breathing

LOW BACK

- Low back pain
- Muscle spasms
- Stiff low back
- Arthritis
- Disc problems, such as herniated discs
- Arthritis in the lower back
- Decreased movement of the lower back
- Pain down the thigh to the knee or the foot (pain may originate below knee)

ABDOMEN (WHEN YOU ARE PASSING MORE GAS THAN A PREGNANT WOMAN EXPECTING TRIPLETS)

- Gas
- Nausea
- Constipation
- Cramping
- Discomfort after eating
- Fatigue after eating
- Loss of appetite
- Diarrhea
- Crohn's disease
- Irritable bowel syndrome (IBS)
- Heartburn
- Gluten intolerance/allergies
- Menstrual pain
- Cramping
- Irregularity
- Heavy cycles
- Abdominal pain
- Irritated stomach
- Abnormal pap smears
- Ovarian cysts
- Infertility
- Impotence
- Inability to have an orgasm

HIPS/LEGS/FEET (HONEY, NO ONE IS RUNNING A MARATHON AROUND HERE ANYTIME SOON.)

- Pain in buttocks
- Pain in one or both hips

- Pain in one or both legs
- Knee pain/problems (even diagnosed arthritis)
- Pain in one or both ankles
- Pain in one or both feet
- Feeling of walking on "broken glass"
- Numbness in either (or both) leg(s)
- Numbness in either (or both) foot (feet)
- Numb toes
- Cold feet (not the kind you get before getting married)
- Burning in either foot
- Cramps in your legs or feet
- Swollen ankles
- Swollen feet
- Pain in toes
- Restless legs
- "Creepy-crawly" feeling in legs at night
- If you are a female, extreme pain may be experienced while shaving your legs. One of my patients described it as a feeling similar to a razor being dragged over a thin layer of broken glass.

ALL THE OTHER ICKY SYMPTOMS

- Suicidal feelings
- Depression
- Anxiety
- Panic attacks
- Nervousness
- Irritability
- Loss of periods of time
- Memory loss
- Fogginess
- Forgetfulness
- Pain during or after exercise

- Cardiac abnormalities
- Pain when it rains or if the weather changes
- Intolerance to heat
- Intolerance to cold
- Intolerance to the wind
- Skin rashes, ranging from the mild- to deep-open wounds that won't heal
- Hair loss
- Bladder pain
- Urinary incontinence
- Feeling of constant fullness in the bladder
- Pain upon urination
- Interstitial cystitis (chronic inflammation of the bladder wall)
- Pain during sexual intercourse or decreased libido
- "Creepy-crawly" feelings all over, or "lightning bolts" of pain
- Insomnia
- Waking up a lot
- Sleep apnea
- Intense, chronic, relentless fatigue (when you don't care if the house burns down to the ground around you—you can't get off your couch)
- Vaginal pain/burning
- Disturbing dreams
- Complete absence of dreams

How is it possible that the long laundry list above, seemingly listing so many things that may possibly plague the human body, could be connected to CRPS? It is easier to understand once you come to realize that CRPS is linked to a global failure of the central nervous system,[6] as demonstrated by quite a few studies.[7] Think of your central nervous system as the commander that runs your entire body, or the power supply to a building. If the main power supply to the building fails, none of your appliances will work. Yet, it would be foolish to try and take apart the toaster or computer, for instance, to see why it is malfunctioning. As we all know, when the less tech savvy of us call for IT support, the first thing we are asked to do is to make sure that our computer is plugged into a power source. If the central nervous system fails, it gives rise to a myriad of problems manifesting in all sorts of symptoms. It may affect nerves, muscles, organs and systems. It may also interfere with the way your body is supposed to function and respond to its environment.

It may also be very reasonable to bring up the fact at this point that many people who do not suffer from CRPS will often suffer from a lot of the symptoms mentioned above. While this is true, the first criteria one must meet in order to be diagnosed with CRPS is mentioned in the beginning of this chapter. Any symptom that you may suffer from in addition should at least be expected to possibly be connected to central nervous system failure that is undeniably linked to CRPS.

I hope that this chapter helped you to make a bit of sense of all your puzzling symptoms. That being said, you really have to get to know your own body. If any symptoms are new, out of the ordinary, or alarming, do not hesitate to see your doctor. It is entirely possible for you to develop a symptom (or symptoms) that signal(s) that something else is wrong with your health. Do not make the mistake of brushing *all* of your symptoms under the CRPS rug. Most importantly, do not allow your doctor to do this, either. When it comes to your health, always, always follow your gut and be diligent. Remember, you alone are responsible for your health. With this realization comes great freedom, as well as great responsibility.

3

You Are Not an Island: How CRPS Affects the Lives of Those Around You

Time was passing like a hand waving from a train I wanted to be on. I hope you never have to think about anything as much as I think about you.

—Jonathan Safran Foer

"It doesn't happen all at once," said the Skin Horse. "You become. It takes a long time. That's why it doesn't happen often to people who break easily, or have sharp edges, or who have to be carefully kept. Generally, by the time you are Real, most of your hair has been loved off, and your eyes drop out and you get loose in the joints and very shabby. But these things don't matter at all, because once you are Real you can't be ugly, except to people who don't understand."

—Margery Williams, The Velveteen Rabbit

YOU DID NOT CHOOSE THIS

A common emotion that I have noticed all CRPS patients share to a greater or lesser degree is guilt. Patients feel guilty for a variety of reasons. They often feel guilty because they feel that they have so little to contribute to all their relationships. They also feel guilty because of the money that has been spent through the years in an attempt to first find a diagnosis, and then relief.

They feel guilty when their health affects their family members' lives and activities. They feel guilty when they can't hug their children, can't make love to their spouse, cannot work, and often feel that they are a constant drain on their families' financial and emotional resources.

The thing about guilt is, it truly doesn't fix anything. It only eats at you from the inside like an acid and at night, when everyone else is asleep, it lies to you and whispers to you that yes, truly, your family would be better off without you. It would be so insensitive of me, a person who has been healthy all her life, to try to convince you that life is good despite your pain and that butterflies and rainbows are to be found in your every day. You live in a hell the likes of which only other people who have walked (or limped) in your shoes can truly understand. Life is not good every day. Frankly, some days it must be hard to remember why you need to go on, and other days just plain suck.

Through the years, however, I have come to know a few great truths: You are alive today because your job here on earth is not done, plain and simple. If you truly could not contribute anything good anymore, I spiritually believe that it would be time for you to go, and that too would be all right in its great divine time. However, here you are. Alive, if not living. Breathing, if not thriving. You *must* figure out why you are still here. What do you have to give? What haven't you learned yet? What is left in life for you, and what do you have left to give others? Another truth is this: most of you do not realize how much you would be missed. You would be missed not as perfect you, healthy you, but *you*. Just the way you are, with your pain, your tough days, your moodiness, your neediness, your desperation, and your disease.

> *Service to others is the rent you pay for your room here on earth.*
>
> —Muhammad Ali

Earlier this year my beloved mother-in-law passed away after many months of a debilitating and dignity-robbing illness. I watched this incredible strong, proud human whither and suffer, and often heard her say; "you guys would be better off if I were gone." The thing is, we aren't better off. Yes, I loved her when she was healthy, painting our toenails together on my in-laws' beautiful back porch, or telling me hilarious stories about my husband's illustrious childhood. However, I also loved her when she was sick. What I would give to have her back even for just one day, so we could visit and I could kiss her cheek and she could hold our babies.

You are loved too. Exactly the way you are. Most people are not islands. When we love and we are loved in return, we are charged with a great responsibility. We form attachments and anchors here on earth binding us irrevocably to our loved ones. We impact their lives and they impact ours. They need us and they learn from us and when we go, we take a piece of them with us, so that they can never truly be whole like before again. You have to remember why your life matters. Broken as you are, you are here. If you can only kiss your grandchild on the cheek once today, you made his or her life better. If you could only watch a small part of a movie with your family tonight, you made your home warmer. If you could pet your dog just for a minute, you made its day. You are unique, an original, and you cannot be replaced.

THE DAY THE MUSIC DIES: CRPS (AKA THE SUICIDE DISEASE)

Let them think what they liked, but I didn't mean to drown myself. I meant to swim till I sank…but that's not the same thing.

—Joseph Conrad

And he suddenly knew that if she killed herself, he would die. Maybe not immediately, maybe not with the same blinding rush of pain, but it would happen. You couldn't live for very long without a heart.

—Jodi Picoult

It is difficult to find exact statistics on CRPS and suicide rates. However, through my years of working with CRPS, I have come across this on CRPS support groups as well as Facebook a heartbreaking number of times. Ninety percent of my CRPS patients have admitted to me that at one point or the other, the thought of ending it all crossed their mind at least once. The thing about chronic pain is that it tends to drive you a little nutty over time. It makes problems seem larger than life; it causes depression, and it wears down your defenses. The truth is though, should you decide to end your life, you will leave behind a legacy of pain that you cannot begin to comprehend. While I am personally in favor of people with painful terminal diseases being allowed to choose to pass on in a humane manner of their own choosing, this should only be an option when all other options have been exhausted, in end-of-life situations. In my opinion, and as thoroughly discussed in this book, CRPS is *not* a hopeless disease.

It is my firm belief that in addition to medical support, every CRPS patient as well as their close family members need emotional support. While family and also individual counseling can prove invaluable, it is not always within everyone's financial reach. However, support may come in many different shapes and forms. Once again, the Internet can prove to be an indispensable tool. In order to receive help, you must reach out and ask for it. No matter what stage of hardship you are in, there will always be someone who has been there, done that. People are usually very willing to help if only you ask.

In addition, your family members may reach out to other family members in the same position they are in. Further on in this chapter, we will discuss family relationships in more detail. However, before we move on to the next topic, I *have* to make sure that you truly hear me in your heart when I say this: Please reach out to someone the moment you find yourself considering even for a moment the possibility of ending your life.

Thoughts are like your mind taking a walk. The first time you think a thought, you are cutting a new path across unchartered neurologic fields. Every time you subsequently think that thought, you are forming a footpath that eventually becomes a broad paved road. This road becomes familiar over time, easier and easier to travel on. Do not allow this to happen to you. Do not allow yourself to make a decision that you can never take back when the proverbial night is at its darkest and you are all alone and your thoughts are driven by screaming pain. Those around you who you will leave behind depend on you for their very happiness and sanity to *not walk down that road*.

National US Suicide Prevention Hotline: 1-800-273-8255. Anytime, 24/7.

Go to www.suicide.org/international-suicide-hotlines.html for international suicide prevention hotlines listed by country.

LOVING SOMEONE WHO SUFFERS FROM CRPS: WHAT IT'S LIKE TO FEEL LIKE COLLATERAL DAMAGE

When you are in a relationship with someone who suffers from chronic pain every day, your life changes in some pretty profound ways. The focus of your entire relationship shifts the moment your partner falls ill. No longer do you get to focus on the usual things nor work toward your old goals. Right off the bat, obtaining first a diagnosis, and then relief, pretty much takes over your lives. Together with this, financial strain will often become overwhelming. Not only do you face mounting medical bills, but often, also a partner who is now unable to contribute financially.

Guilt becomes your constant and silent companion. The person in pain feels guilty for all the reasons mentioned earlier in this chapter. In addition to feeling like a financial drain, daily pain tends to erode your identity as a man or a woman. When you are no longer able to do things for your spouse, to contribute financially nor physically to your daily household chores or parenting, you start to question your self-worth. What do you bring to your relationship? Your self-confidence slips. Why would anyone want to be tied to me? Am I still even sexy? Am I still attractive? Am I still wanted?

Being the other half of this couple is tough too. When we take those "for better or for worse, through sickness and in health" vows, no one envisions a future that may include CRPS. It is easy to be understanding, supportive, and loving if your partner has the flu or is involved in a car accident. The circumstances may not be ideal, but the story has an end. You know that after feeding them some chicken soup and doing some pampering your partner will recover and you will have them back the way they were before.

However, if your partner suffers from CRPS, the future is bleak by all accounts. The pain is daily, chronic, relentless, and it renders you helpless. You are leaned on pretty heavily, and you do get fatigued. It gets old, always having to be understanding, sympathetic, and strong. When you get frustrated, you may beat yourself up. Partners often feel that they don't have the right to get overwhelmed nor frustrated. Sure, life dealt you an unfair hand, but at least you are not in daily pain, right? You watch your partner suffer and you feel so darn *guilty* for feeling tired, angry, cheated or resentful. You miss your partner the way he or she used to be. You may miss your fun times, his or her laughter, your dreams of the future, and your old sex life. If you have children, you become like a single parent in many ways. Your heart aches for the parent that your kids are missing out on. The whole thing is complicated and heartbreaking. However, nothing can exist in darkness only.

> *One word frees us of all the weight and pain of life: That word is love.*
>
> —S<small>OPHOCLES</small>

Learning to love each other despite the unwelcome third partner that is daily chronic pain is not an easy task, but it is possible. I have seen it in my practice. Love is a beautiful, wonderful thing. The force of true love cannot ever be underestimated. Where there is love, the seed of greatness always exist. A relationship that has been forged in a fire becomes stronger and tough and able to weather all. You must find a way to recognize that love every single day. It is my spiritual belief that we are brought together by forces greater than us.

When we set out on a journey together, we do not know which obstacles we will face. We don't know our road. All we can do is to believe that the road we are on has a purpose and lessons and blessings of its own which we cannot always understand in the moment. Hope, faith and love carry us through. As a couple, you are stronger than you will ever know, until you have the chance to discover your own strengths. Having studied successful and loving couples who have coped and survived the pain of CRPS, I am astounded at what is possible in the face of love. Patients have told me that while they would never wish the pain of CRPS upon anyone, they would not give back the gifts or blessings that surviving it together has given them.

In the meantime, you must both view yourselves much like electric appliances that need to be recharged from time to time. While leaning on each other can be a beautiful thing, you must also sometimes move away from each other in order to briefly recharge. This way, when you come back together, you will have more to give in addition to renewed strength. "Charging" may come in many shapes or forms. Friends, family, time apart or support groups are all very valuable tools. The healthy partner needs loving support just as much as the sick partner does. Do not ever underestimate the power of recharging your battery.

I am a very big proponent of ongoing counseling. Ideally, counseling should be individual as well as in the form of couples counseling. Our worst fears are sometimes dispelled just being able to verbalize it to a third party. Every couple faces tough times and communication problems at least at some point. Couples dealing with CRPS face more obstacles than most. Every ounce of extra support is needed. Facing any hardship together is easier than facing it alone. You guys can do this. It is a fact. It has been done by many others.

HEARTBREAK AT ITS WORST: WHEN YOU AREN'T ABLE TO BE THE PARENT YOU WANT TO BE

Guilt takes on a whole new meaning once your children are involved. It is a sad fact that CRPS is so intense by nature, that it inadvertently will also touch your children's lives. Even being a healthy parent can be tough, and will naturally always be accompanied by some guilt. As humans, we are going to make mistakes. Sometimes, those mistakes will affect our children. Our children will sometimes be forced to grow up faster than we would have liked for them. Just as we do not always get to pick our own circumstances, we do not get to pick our children's circumstances either. Please remember that ultimately, your most important task as a parent is to love your child wholly and completely. CRPS may rob you of your smiles, your energy, and your ability to physically participate in your children's lives. The one thing it cannot take from you, however, and that can never be underestimated, is love.

When I catch myself feeling riddled by guilt about dragging my son through a divorce, I always think back to a conversation I once had with one of my very wise mentors. He told me that we do not ever know what our children's lives are supposed to look like. We often hold on to an ideal that we build up in our minds. This ideal usually involves strong, happy, secure families and our children not having to suffer any significant heartbreak if we can help it. We assume that our children should not suffer disappointment, abandonment, loneliness, or hard times. We love them so deeply, so purely, that we would gladly lay down our lives for them. We want their worlds to be perfect in ways that ours weren't.

However, life was not meant to always be easy, not even if you are just a kid. The life we want for our kids may not be the life they had chosen in order to forge them into the adults they will one day become. We do not know what hardships today may serve them tomorrow, and truthfully, it is not our job to know. Our job is simple and direct—we must love them. No one can love your child more than you can. No one can replace you in this one important task. Even when you are physically or mentally absent due to pain, your love for your child is always there, and they know this. Know that it is normal to feel guilt, but that every parent feels guilt sooner or later anyway.

Think about life on earth as a blessing, but also an obstacle course, meant to make us stronger, tougher, wiser, more interesting, more loving, more understanding, and more resilient. Some of the greatest people in history grew up in very tough circumstances. Oprah Winfrey, Jim Carrey, Helen Keller, Tina Turner, Gloria Steinem, and Tyler Perry are just a few famous people who overcame incredibly difficult childhoods only to become successful later on in life. It is the belief of many spiritual people and also myself that we play a role in selecting our lives, our parents, and our circumstances for reasons not always immediately known. While you may not subscribe to this belief, you must at least be able to see that every dark cloud inevitably has a silver lining, and even the toughest lessons leave us with more wisdom after.

Once again, it is very important that every family coping with daily chronic pain suffered by one of its members should seek counseling and support in some form. It is very important that your children know that they are not to blame for the increased difficulties your family faces. Please know that you don't have to be perfect or healthy as long as you love your child. Nobody can do that better than you. I bet that one day, when your child is an adult and looks back, he or she would still choose to have had you around, exhausted and in pain, rather than not having had you around at all.

Just do the best you can. Surround yourself with a strong support network that can pick up the slack where your health forces you to fall short sometimes. You don't have to be a perfect healthy parent. What matters is being there at night to tuck them in and tell them you love them. Explain that sometimes you hurt, but that everything is going to be OK, that you are doing your best, and that you love them and always will.

If you have a significant other, understand that if your roles were reversed, you would be the primary practical caregiver. Let them be that, and you focus on just doing the best you can, while still being gentle with your sick body. When people offer to help you, accept their help. You deserve support where and when you can get it. Your children deserve it also. Do not try to be a superhero. Allow your child to help you in small ways. This may be as simple as just bringing you a glass of water or giving you a hug. While you may not want your child to become your nurse, it is important that your child learns at a young age that we help to take care of and support those we love who are in need. Make sure that you explain your condition openly and honestly to your child. This will help them to understand your limitations and also to not take it personal. Open and honest communication is vital. Your child needs to understand that while you are hurting, you are not dying, and they do not have to be afraid for you. Security is very important to children of all ages.

THE HORROR OF WATCHING THE MONSTER ATTACK YOUR CHILD

I want to acknowledge one of the groups of people affected by CRPS the most—parents of children with CRPS. It doesn't matter if your baby is two years old or fifty-three. As a mother myself, I think the only pain worse than CRPS is watching your child suffer from CRPS.

My phone calls with you, brave parents, both horrify me and inspire me. You tell me stories of endless suffering. Stories of your daughter missing her prom, and of your son never being able to walk on to a baseball field. Stories of your children crawling instead of walking, and of their days in bed, as you watch their friends play sports, go to school, date, and move on to college. At night you worry about their future. Will they find love, careers, and have babies. Who will watch over them when you are gone.

Your lives are not understood well except by other CRPS parents. Your misery is an island, unfathomable by most. How can anyone understand what it feels like to watch your child burn alive every day?

You give me your children's medical history in a matter-of-fact way with military precision, which tells me you've done it a hundred times before. You don't want my pity. You've put up a wall that rejects pity like a dam wall holds in water, for if this wall should crack, your sorrow may drown you. You cannot afford to drown. You are fighting for your child, and you can't, won't, give up. You will spend every penny you have fighting, because this is your baby. You were charged with protecting them.

My God, do I admire you. You did not choose this, I know, but you are surviving it day by difficult day. You are the pillar that your child leans against, and you stand strong so they can do so. I admire every part of what you do with every part of me. You are the reason I know that this is the most important thing I will ever do in my career.

As a parent, I cannot imagine a more horrific hand to be dealt by life than to be forced to stand by helplessly while your child suffers from daily, unimaginable pain. Please allow me to say that my heart goes out to you. I cannot imagine anything more difficult. As a parent, we want only what is best for our children. It is our *job* to protect them. We do everything in our power to make sure that our children are safe, happy and protected. However, sometimes, life will present them with circumstances beyond our control and our sheer willpower. CRPS is one of those circumstances.

As a parent of a child who suffers daily, you have only one true choice: You must become an asset to your child. This will require incredible strength and willpower, sometimes under very difficult circumstances. While it is normal to want to scream at the heavens "why?" at the top of your lungs, it won't ultimately change a thing. CRPS cannot be kissed away by a parent's love. However, by becoming steadfast and informed, you will be a strong pillar for your child that they may hold on to during the worst of storms.

When my niece Mia was born, she suffered from a genetic condition that affected, among other things, her heart. At the tender age of five weeks, Mia had to undergo open-heart surgery. My sister Hannelie, also a physician, taught me incredible life lessons during this time. Her husband, due to immigration laws at the time, was stuck in South Africa, and she faced all of this on her own. I watched my sister rise to this occasion with incredible pride and admiration that I hold in my heart like a pearl of wisdom to this day. She never cried where we could see her. She used every ounce of fear and doubt and transformed it into strength instead. She viewed Mia's health problems as an obstacle that she would overcome for the sake of her child. She always focused on every positive moment in every day.

After Mia's surgery, she made it her task to understand the monstrous medical machinery that kept her little girl alive just as well as the nurses did. In this, she found her strength and her will to fight for her child. To this day, this is how she handles obstacles involving her children. While I tend to overprotect, my sister views every challenge as a potential source of strength for her child. While she is incredibly loving, she never allows any physical limitation to become an excuse. She taught Mia to face every challenge with the same gusto and sheer willpower. As a result, Mia has turned into a little warrior. She is confident, happy, and spunky. I believe that my sister had (and has) a lot to do with this.

While your child will need to cry on your shoulder sometimes, you cannot allow yourself to collapse into a puddle of pity at those times. Your child needs to feel secure in a world that is made very insecure by the very nature of CRPS. They will look to you for strength when they are in pain, doubtful, in a state of self-pity, angry, and scared. You will be their constant port as they are caught in a storm they cannot control. Yes, love them always. Cradle them always. However, you must understand that your child needs you to fight for them. They need for you to be strong when they can't be. Once again, please find sources of energy and support, that will allow you to "plug in" when you become overwhelmed. While it is important to be able to be honest with your child, you need to hold on to your strength so that your child never has to see you fall apart.

Children who deal with daily chronic pain feel acute guilt because of the effect that their condition has on the entire family. It is very important that you tell your child that even though they are not physically perfect as far as their health is concerned, that this does not change how much their sheer existence contributes to your life, as well as that of the rest of the family. They have to know that they still matter in many meaningful ways. This is where counseling becomes incredibly valuable, not only for them, but also for your marriage or relationship, as well as your relationship with your child's siblings. While your family will face more obstacles than most, these obstacles can be overcome and at the end of the day, leave your family stronger than before. I know you can do this. Do you know why? Your child chose you. They were born into this world through you. Their souls saw strength in you that therefore must exist. They picked you to be their parent, and in that choice bestowed an incredible privilege upon you.

> *Your children are not your children. They are the sons and daughters of Life's longing for itself. They come through you but not from you. And though they are with you, yet they belong not to you.*
>
> —Kahlil Gibran

4

The Perfect Storm: How You Got Sick

Knowing yourself is the beginning of all wisdom.

—Aristotle

Yesterday is gone. Tomorrow has not yet come. We have only today. Let us begin.

—Mother Teresa

What causes CRPS? This is probably one of the most burning questions among patients who suffer from CRPS. I have found that patients have come to expect a very succinct answer to this question. They are looking for that one abnormal genetic fingerprint, that one explanation (it is an autoimmune condition! It is a brain abnormality!) that will finally explain it all. The reasoning, of course, is that once they find the cause, they can find a cure.

The logic with this thinking is clear and understandable. You have a health problem that is dominating your life, and you need a solution. The error in this way of thinking is that most diseases or conditions do not simply have one single, simple cause. The body is not simple, it is incredibly complex. CRPS is no exception. In my opinion, what leads to the development of CRPS is much like a perfect storm. A whole bunch of unfortunate circumstances combine to give rise to this monstrous disease. While it is complicated, it is by no means impossible to unravel. It is my true belief that in order to understand CRPS and find any long-term successful treatment, you must first have a clear understanding of *why* you got sick. In order to understand how your body got into trouble, you must understand how the body works. Most patients today have been indoctrinated by current modern mechanistic thinking when it comes to health. Please allow me to explain.

MECHANISTIC VERSUS VITALISTIC APPROACHES TO SYMPTOM TREATING AND HEALING
The Mechanistic View

This view, which dominates health care in the United States and most of the world today, tends to ignore the *cause* of the illness or condition. Its focus is primarily symptom-based. Think of your body as a car. It is made up of parts. When your car won't start one morning, it is taken or towed to the mechanic, where the part or parts most likely causing the specific problem are examined and replaced if necessary. The alternator may be broken, but the rest of the car still works. Therefore, the alternator is fixed or replaced. This is how mechanistic health care works. The body is viewed as a machine where one part has nothing to do with the other, and organs and systems may be tested and treated independently of other organs and symptoms. I hesitate to even call this model "health care." It is focused mainly on "disease care" and, more specifically, on emergency care.

What do I mean by this? In traditional health care today, "preventative" care is virtually nonexistent, and what is passed off as such truly should be labeled as *early detection* instead. For example, once a year, most women past a certain age are urged to undergo breast exams, mammograms and pelvic exams, all geared to detect cancer or other problems early. The same rings true for men and prostate exams. The body is typically ignored—except for periodically being tested and examined for problems by your doctor—until a sign or symptom of malfunction rears its ugly head. At this point, you make an appointment to see your doctor and the symptom is examined, diagnosed, and managed. The focus of all treatments seems to be symptom-oriented—isolate the broken or malfunctioning body part or organ guided by symptoms, fix it or numb it with surgery or medications, or remove the offending part(s).

The philosophy is a simple one—if there is pain, numb it. If the patient is not sleeping at night, force their body to sleep at night by drugging it. If the patient has pain somewhere, give them painkillers. If they appear to also suffer from, let's say, irritable bowel syndrome (IBS), the relationship between these two sets of symptoms is seldom examined and tend to be treated separately. The patient will be given a thorough exam and probably go through some tests, and in the end, a different doctor will most likely manage the IBS with different medications. Doctors specialize in their unique fields, and communication between doctors leaves much to be desired. In addition, we are bombarded with ads for designer medications for every condition under the sun. Have you heard these words lately while watching your favorite show? "Ask your doctor about…" The message is clear: manage every symptom. Squash it, numb it, interrupt it, silence it, or cut it out.

If the mechanistic way of doing things worked, it is obvious that the United States would be full of healthy people. We have some of the best hospitals, the best doctors, and more pharmaceutical companies than you can throw a rock at. A good example of this is the great American tradition of direct-to-consumer advertising, where drugs are marketed directly to the public. You know the ads. It typically goes like this—attractive actors, celebrities, and cartoons (ever seen the bee that is voiced by Antonio Banderas?) ask you if you suffer from a list of symptoms. You do? Well, presto! They have the answer in the form of some drug. This is followed by members of the public being urged to "ask their doctor" about the drug by name, finally followed by a long list of side effects rambled off very rapidly, resembling a witch's book of spells. (Bleeding from the nose?)

Drug companies like Pfizer spend around six billion dollars a year on this type of marketing. The nation's health-care tab is on a fast track to hit approximately $4.6 trillion in 2020, accounting for about $1 of every $5 in the economy.[8] Our brains have a tendency to skip over complicated statements that contain large numbers. However, make sure that you understand that this holds vast complications for all of us. In theory, if everyone in the United States should become even 50 percent healthier overnight, our economy would literally collapse. There is big money in disease. This is not a conspiracy theory, it is a fact.

The largest profits do not come from healthy people or dead people, but from the chronically ill. Most medical research today is funded by the pharmaceutical industry. The pharmaceutical industry is much like your local drug dealer on the corner, only, much, much more powerful. The pharmaceutical industry is incredibly powerful because it is backed by so much money. Between 1998 and 2015, more money (about 3.2 billion) was spent on lobbying by the pharmaceutical industry than any other. Coming in second (and lagging behind by about one billion) is the insurance industry. Drug companies make laws, and medical research is not driven by compassion nor a desire to find a cure for diseases and conditions. It is driven by money. There is no money in the cure. We *must* stop being naïve and realize that the only one who really, truly care about you becoming healthy, is you and those you love. The buck stops with you.

Let's get back to the mechanistic approach. Are Americans healthier because of it? Not exactly. A new report done in 2013 prepared by a panel of doctors, epidemiologists, and other researchers at the request of the National Research Council and the Institute of Medicine, found a "strikingly consistent and pervasive" pattern of poorer health of Americans at all stages of life. In fact, Americans' health ranked below that of sixteen other developed nations. We may live longer than we used to, but what is the quality of those extended lives? As you can attest, living with chronic daily pain is really not a picnic. It is agony.

The Vitalistic View

The vitalistic viewpoint takes a very different approach. The body is seen as more than the sum of its parts. It is understood that the body is a masterful, intelligent system where every part affects every other part. It is studied in terms of its dynamic connections with its environment. It boils down to: fix the whole, including its environment, and the parts will take care of themselves.

When we study the body by looking at smaller and smaller parts, we may find certain organs or systems that are not working properly. For example, a patient may suffer from diabetes if the pancreas isn't producing insulin. However, the *cause* of the pancreas not producing insulin is rarely addressed. When a giant corporation finds itself in hot water for some reason, blame is usually not laid at the feet of each individual worker all the way down to the mailroom and cleaning staff. Rather, the top management of the company is scrutinized first, together with its policies. In much the same way, it makes more sense to examine a malfunctioning body from the top down. View the body as a corporation where the brain and spinal cord form the central nervous system (CNS); that is the CEO.

YOUR AMAZING BODY

I often ask patients whether they appreciate how incredibly intelligent their bodies are. This is often met with scorn and annoyance by those with less-than-stellar health. People who suffer from CRPS often have a sense that their bodies have betrayed them in some way. They feel as if they can't trust their bodies, since those very bodies have let them down. It is a source of pain, and it keeps them from doing the things they love, which is understandable. But let's step back for a moment and look at this differently. The body of a patient who suffers from CRPS is under immense ongoing stress. It doesn't have the life-giving energy available to it that normal people have. Each cell is functioning under stress. Yet it chugs on like the little engine that could. It is essential that you regain a sense of love and respect for this amazing living organism that allows you to live another day, as this is part of the recovery process.

Do you think your body isn't all it's cracked up to be? Let's look at some of the things this body of yours can do. Your body was designed to survive (sometimes horrific) injuries even if a large part of your internal organs was removed. The human body may appear fragile, but it's possible to survive even with the removal of the stomach, the spleen, 75 percent of the liver, 80 percent of the intestines, one kidney, one lung, and virtually every organ from the pelvic and groin area. You might not feel too great, but the missing organs wouldn't kill you.

Your body is innately intelligent. It does many, many things at once. If I asked you to consciously and accurately monitor your blood pressure, heart rate, blood sugar levels, and temperature for ten minutes, it would be impossible to do so without the help of some serious technology. Yet your body does this and more every millisecond of every day and night without your having to give it any thought. We can think of the human body as an organized collection of infinitely intelligent cells. Each cell is like an elaborate biochemical computer. It has its own power-management and information-processing structures. It continuously communicates with its neighbors and the environment.

Each cell is an individual organism. Under certain conditions it may even be capable of living outside of the body. Most cells have a complete copy of the body's genetic information and are theoretically capable of recreating the whole human body. The magnitude of information-processing activity inside the human body is amazing. The cell reproduction processes require terabytes of genetic information to be copied every second within the body. And the protein formation and other functions in cells can be several orders of magnitude more information-intensive. The power consumption of a single cell corresponds to about 10^7 chemical reactions per second.

The smartest scientist in the world cannot create life from scratch, or a hair from nothing. Your body serves you well. You may be thinking that while all this information is nifty, it does not explain why your body somehow became messed up and now has you feeling like dog poop every day. Nor does it explain why it's not repairing itself already. This is a valid point! As one of my patients once so eloquently put it: "awesome body my behind Dr. K!" I understood her frustration just like I understand yours.

There has to be a reason *why* this supposedly amazing, self-healing and self-regulating body of yours has gone on the fritz. Let's look at why this happens.

THAT OVERUSED WORD: STRESS

> *Where'd the days go, when all we did was play? And the stress that we were under wasn't stress at all just a run and jump into a harmless fall.*
>
> —Paolo Nutini

My dad, who is one of my greatest mentors and has been a chiropractor for forty-one years, likes to tell his patients that their stress will end the day the lid on their coffin is closed. What he means by this is that stress is an unavoidable part of human existence. We can no more avoid stress than we can avoid breathing. However, once you understand that it is not stress *itself* that makes us sick, it may bring you some peace and comfort. Who wants to be a victim of stress? Wouldn't you rather be the one in control? The good news is that you *are* in control.

We usually think of stress as all bad, but that is not necessarily true. Let's look at what stress *actually* is. The official definition of stress in medicine isthe result produced when a stressor (something or someone) causes stress to a structure, system, or organism. When stress occurs in quantities that the system cannot handle, it produces pathological changes. In layperson's terms, stress technically is *any* change that requires your body to change in order to process it. If you follow this logic, even eating a banana can cause the body stress. If you didn't swallow it and it became stuck in your throat, it could suffocate you, resulting in your untimely demise. In addition, if your body could not digest and eliminate it, it would make you very sick. Although we typically associate stress with an emotional upset, there are actually three kinds of stress that affect your health—physical, chemical, and emotional stress.

PHYSICAL STRESS

Physical stress comes from the world outside of your body. A car accident is an excellent example of a physical stress that may contribute to a patient's developing CRPS. Patients will often tell me that although they had a car accident, it was insignificant and could not have caused significant injuries to their necks because they (or the car that hit them) were driving really slowly when it happened and there was little damage to their vehicles. Sometimes they think it's not worth mentioning during their history since it happened a long time ago. Please note that *the force of the impact or the time that has gone by since the injury often has no effect on the extent of the injury.*

One researcher has shown that when a thirty-five hundred–pound car traveling at ten miles an hour strikes the rear of another car, it may transmit to this car a force of twenty-five tons. The person in the car that is struck continues to move forward while his or her head, being hinged at the neck, snaps backward. The average head weighs about eight pounds, and the cervical vertebrae (the bones of the neck) are very delicate; the force pushing the head backward is even greater than you might believe since the base of the neck acts as a fulcrum and the leverage is applied near the top of the head.

Therefore, the head snaps back with the equivalent of several tons of force without any support, since the muscle control of the neck is caught off guard. The end result, with the neck in acute hyperextension, is that the nerve root (where the nerve exits the spinal cord) is caught in a pincer between the superior and inferior facets (the special posterior joints of the spine).[9] Car accidents are not the only culprits. The cervical spine may be injured in a number of different ways—falls, birth injuries, long-forgotten childhood injuries, sports injuries, or any injuries that caused you to suffer a concussion or cervical spine (neck) injury.

Another way patients may be injured is through general anesthesia. When the muscles that normally hold the bones of the neck in a safe position are paralyzed by the anesthesia, it is easy for the neck to be injured, especially if the neck is bent back in order for the breathing tube to be inserted in the patient's throat. Injuries to the neck are so prevalent in patients who suffer from CRPS that we will devote more space to the neck and nervous system elsewhere in this book.

Other examples of physical injuries include injuries to the cranial nerves (the nerves that control your senses, like hearing, sight, and smell). I have a patient (let's call her Bonnie) who was doing very well after her third month of treatment. Her big goal after recovery was to go to Florida on a vacation with a girlfriend. After a trip to an amusement park, where she went on some of the spinning rides, she suffered severe nausea and dizziness for a month after returning home. The cranial nerves dealing with her balance had been injured. Such injuries can also be caused by excessive visual or auditory stimulation. (Interestingly enough, she underwent several needless, grueling tests ordered by her MDs targeting her digestive system before she finally happened to mention to me one day that her nausea had started *immediately* following the ride at the amusement park.)

The body was designed to heal after injuries. However, sometimes the body is already under stress at the time of a physical injury, making it harder to recover afterward. Think how much easier it is for a string to snap if it is pulled very taut. For example, let's say that you are going through a divorce. One night you are particularly upset. You are driving home after an emotionally wrenching day that ended with a nasty phone call from your soon-to-be ex, and then to top it all off, you are hit from behind by another car. The fact that you were under emotional stress at the time of the accident, causing your body to be tense, will make it much more likely that you will be injured by that car accident and make it more difficult to recover.

During a traumatic event, the nervous system goes into survival mode (exciting or turning on the sympathetic nervous system) and sometimes has difficulty reverting back into its normal, relaxed mode again (controlled by the parasympathetic nervous system). If your nervous system is stuck in survival mode, stress hormones such as cortisol are constantly released, causing an increase in blood pressure and blood sugar, which can in turn reduce the immune system's ability to heal. Physical symptoms start to manifest when the body is in constant distress. If you add a physical injury on top of these conditions, the body now enters a danger zone where healing does not occur as easily as it should.

CHEMICAL STRESS

We are blessed with free choice. Every day, we get to choose the things we eat and drink. Your body responds to every single thing you put into it, whether you swallow it, inject it, rub it on your skin, or inhale it. After it enters our bodies, the part of us that gets to choose, however, is no longer in control. Now it is up to your body to process what you just put into it. Did it add to your health, or take away from it? Elsewhere in this book, we will devote an entire chapter to nutrition and supplements. For now, nutrition deserves to be briefly mentioned. Food will either enhance your health or take away from it.

Medications can add tremendous stress to the already stressed body of a CRPS patient. It is very important for every CRPS patient who is taking a lot of medications to support their liver and kidneys with detoxification and nutritional supplements.

Another bad habit that many people in chronic pain cling to is smoking. You'd have to live under a rock to not know that smoking is bad for you. It is especially detrimental to those who suffer from CRPS because it decreases oxygen to the brain and increases neurological injury. Alcohol and nicotine add to your toxic chemical load. It should go without saying that these vices are especially detrimental to patients who already suffer from CRPS. Please note that even secondhand smoke, or smoke clinging to the clothes of someone next to you, will affect your brain oxygen levels.

In my experience, it is much harder for a patient to recover from any condition, CRPS included, if they refuse to give up smoking. In addition to putting a tremendous stress on the lungs and decreasing oxygen to the brain, smoking will add toxins like heavy metals to your system that will interfere with your healing. A good example of this is cadmium. Cadmium is an extremely toxic metal commonly found in cigarettes that is very easily absorbed by the lungs. Cadmium may cause osteoporosis, arthritis, kidney pain, and a host of other unpleasant symptoms.

When a smoker enters care, I am decidedly more apprehensive of their recovery than with normal patients, unless the patient is able to undergo the difficult process of quitting smoking. Adding to your toxic load will not help you to feel better or to live a longer, better life. However, we understand that daily pain will sometimes cause people to make poor choices in health. It is very difficult to stop a bad habit that is nevertheless comforting if you are in pain. Judging, we are not. However, you will show your body tremendous love and support if you can stop these bad habits. If necessary, get professional help. I have found that hypnosis is especially helpful in kicking toxic habits, as it addresses not only the physical but also the emotional and powerful subconscious addiction.

DIET SUGARS: JUST GO FOR THE SUGAR IF YOU MUST

I wanted to address diet drinks and sugar separately. Most notably, I want to mention aspartame. Aspartame is the technical name for the brand names Spoonful, NutraSweet, Equal, and Equal-Measure. It was discovered by accident in the sixties when James Schlatter, a chemist, was testing an ulcer drug. Aspartame accounts for over 75 percent of the adverse reactions to food additives reported to the FDA. Many of these reactions are very serious, including seizures and death.

Aspartame is found in almost every single brand of gum, something that patients who suffer from CRPS are particularly fond of in my experience. It is also found in diet sodas and drinks and in many other foods, including some children's vitamins. Recently, the EPA found aspartame to be a potentially dangerous chemical along with BPA (Bisphenol A), which you've no doubt heard a lot about in the news lately. BPA is the harmful chemical that is often released by plastic cups, toys, and containers, especially when heated up. Most parents now know that their baby's bottle should be BPA free. However, have you heard about aspartame being bad for you in mainstream media lately? Not so much.

WHAT IS ASPARTAME MADE OF?

Aspartame is made of three components: 50 percent phenylalanine, 40 percent aspartic acid, and 10 percent methanol (wood alcohol). In the body, methanol breaks down into formaldehyde (embalming fluid) and formic acid. While going through school and doing human dissection, formaldehyde was one of the smells that clung to me and my classmates in a stinky chemical fog that seemed to repel the public. After a while, it is almost impossible to remove the smell from your skin. It is used to preserve cadavers and acts as a preservative inside of the body. Today, our bodies are exposed to so many preservatives that they are actually taking much longer to decay after death. Gross, right? While it used to take a body about eight years to crumble into dust (hence "dust to dust"), it can now take forty years or longer! Maybe it's just me, but I find this fact particularly creepy.

ASPARTIC ACID (40 PERCENT OF ASPARTAME)

Dr. Russell L. Blaylock, a professor of neurosurgery at the University of Mississippi Medical centerpublished a book thoroughly describing the damage caused by the ingestion of too much aspartic acid. He makes use of almost five hundred scientific references to show how excess free amino acids such as aspartic acid and glutamic acid do damage to the human body. Monosodium glutamate (MSG) is the sodium salt of glutamic acid or glutamate. Found in our food supply, it is causing serious chronic neurological disorders and a ton of other unwanted symptoms, such as numbness, vertigo, and seizures.

HOW ASPARTATE (AND GLUTAMATE) CAUSE DAMAGE

Aspartame releases aspartate during digestion. Aspartate and glutamate (MSG is the sodium salt of glutamate) act as neurotransmitters (think of them as chemical taxis) in the brain by facilitating the transmission of information from neuron to neuron. Too much aspartate or glutamate in the brain kills certain neurons by allowing the influx of too much calcium into the cells. This influx triggers excessive amounts of free radicals, which kill the cells. The neural cell damage that can be caused by excessive aspartate and glutamate is why they are referred to as "excitotoxins." They "excite" or stimulate the neural cells to death. My colleagues and I have observed that few things will injure the nervous system as rapidly and completely as aspartame.

Splenda is another culprit. It is marketed in such a savvy way that you would swear it's made by Mother Nature herself. It is often included in products labeled as "all-natural." However, Splenda is chlorinated sugar and is anything but natural. There have been no long-term human studies on the safety of Splenda; however, several issues have been raised about Splenda. According to a study from Duke University, Splenda "suppresses beneficial bacteria and directly affects the expression of the transporter isozymes that are known to interfere with the bioavailability of drugs and nutrients. Furthermore, these effects occur at Splenda doses that contain sucralose levels that are approved by the FDA for use in the food supply."[10]

A great natural alternative is the sweetener stevia, which is derived from a plant. *Stevia* was first discovered in 1500 and widely used for hundreds of years by American Indians. In the early seventies, as problems with other sweeteners emerged, Japan started widely using stevia. Today, it accounts for 40 percent of all sweetened products produced in Japan. Numerous studies in the United States and Europe found stevia to be safe and even beneficial. Your local health-food store should carry this sweetener in its natural form (I recommend the KAL brand). If you chew on a stevia plant leaf, you will find that it is naturally sweet. A great rule of thumb is that the more humans interfere with food, the worse it is for you.

COSMETICS

A large number of personal care and cosmetic products, including deodorants, lotions, makeup, and even baby shampoos, contain chemicals that are linked to cancer, learning disabilities, birth defects, asthma, and other health problems. The average woman today uses about a dozen personal care products daily, containing more than one hundred and twenty chemicals. I like to tell my patients that if you can't eat it, you should not put it on your skin. We forget that the skin is not an impenetrable covering surrounding our bodies, but also a living, breathing organ rich with blood supply that serves as a portal of entry straight into the body.

If you suffer from CRPS, I suggest you take extra care to protect your body from toxic chemicals such as lead (still contained in many lipsticks), phthalates (industrial chemicals contained in almost every cosmetic and personal care product and that have been shown to disrupt the endocrine system), sulfates, heavy metals, and countless other harmful chemicals. A great resource that I recommend to my patients is the Environmental Working Group's "skin deep" website (http://www.ewg.org/skindeep).

EWG's Skin Deep database gives you practical solutions to protect yourself and your family from everyday exposure to chemicals. It was launched in 2004 to create online safety profiles for cosmetics and personal care products. Their aim is to fill in where industry and government leave off. Using this website, you can look up the safety and ingredients of most of the products that you use, and the effects the chemicals contained in these products have on the human body.

That being said, I don't recommend that you obsess about the thousands of chemicals you *can't* avoid. Even babies in utero have been shown to be exposed to harmful chemicals. It is impossible to completely avoid our toxic environment. However, educate yourself on the products that you use daily and make better choices where you can. For example, instead of buying only organic produce, look up the "dirtiest" fruits and vegetables (see chapter 11 for a complete list), and try to buy these only if they are certified organically grown.

It is a good rule of thumb to detoxify the whole body at least quarterly. This can be done in many ways. I like the Isagenix nine-day detoxification, and a *good quality* ionic footbath (not all are created equal). I also like doing this through eating a very pure diet, as described in chapter 11.

EMOTIONAL STRESS

Although we often blame emotional stress on the actions of people around us as well as the ups and downs of life in general, it is actually the one stress completely in our power to control. Emotional stress is nothing more than feelings that don't feel good, originating from our thoughts. Every person has a unique filter through which they experience the world. Whether we experience something as pleasant or unpleasant, good or bad, happy or sad has much to do with our upbringing, our ethical values, and that which we hold dear. I had a mentor who used to tell his patients something I will never forget: "You can spit in my face, but you cannot *make* me mad." We can't control the actions of others. However, we can control the *feelings* their actions cause us to feel.

Close your eyes and "feel" your thoughts for a second. Every thought, if we focus on our bodies, tends to be accompanied by an actual physical sensation; these sensations are generally distinctly pleasant or unpleasant. Close your eyes and focus on a thought. Now pay attention to the physical sensation that thought generates in your body. Is there a nice warm feeling in your chest, about where you imagine your heart is located, or do you have an unpleasant feeling in the pit in your stomach? Does it feel like your heart is being squeezed with fear and dread or that a heavy weight is resting on your chest? Are you feeling boredom, annoyance, terror, or frustration?

EMOTIONAL STRESS AND HOW IT AFFECTS YOUR NERVOUS SYSTEM

Let's imagine that your brain is a computer. You have hardware (brain cells, nerves, white matter, gray matter, the spinal cord, and so on), and software (the signals you can't *see*, but that you know are there). If you decide to pick up a glass of water, your nerves respond to the decision made by the great CEO, the brain. They pass the command down to the muscles of your arm and fingers. These muscles and tendons contract and relax to move the bones, and, presto! You are holding a glass.

You have a conscious mind and a subconscious mind. The conscious mind resides in the cerebral cortex, which is a thin layer of nerve cells about one-eighth of an inch thick that surrounds your brain. The conscious mind is your thinking, judging, and decision-making mind. This is the area we use when we make choices. This area is fed by the five senses (what you see, hear, smell, taste, and feel) and by information entering your mind through the cranial nerves discussed elsewhere in this book. When you learn to ride a bike, that information is programmed in the cerebral cortex where you can access it at any time.

Over time, as your body builds muscle memory and the actions of riding a bike or walking become routine, the knowledge is dumped in the area underneath this layer, the cerebrum. Occasionally, these bits of information may not be easily accessible (e.g., when you forget someone's name). For the most part, however, the information in the conscious mind is readily available. Think of it as the thinking mind, or a vast library of information. When you are born, the conscious mind is a blank slate. As we have our first human experiences as babies, this area is programmed. We may learn that the appearance of our mother's face is shortly followed by comfort and food, and that if we cry, our demands are met. We may also learn useful bits of information. For example: if we touch a hot curling iron or a pan, this brings pain, and it should be avoided for the rest of our life.

The subconscious mind is the area that runs our bodies, driven by one singular, razor-sharp goal: survival. It is the lower "animal" part of our brain at the base of our skull. When we are born, this area is already filled with all we need built-in for survival. The newborn baby does not need to be taught how to regulate his or her insulin, how to digest milk, or how to breathe. This part cannot think, judge, or reason. It simply responds to what is being programmed into the conscious mind.

Imagine that you are driving along one day and notice a police car with flashing lights in your rear-view mirror. You may become scared. Your subconscious or automatic (or autonomic) nervous system will respond by going into survival mode. Your heart rate will go up, your hands may sweat on the steering wheel, and your stomach may pull into a knot. When the police car passes you, you will take a deep breath and laugh about how silly you were. The body usually will take a few minutes to respond, but eventually your heart will slow down, and you may even feel relaxed enough to stop and grab something to eat.

The subconscious mind cannot distinguish between a real threat to your survival and a fake one. It cannot distinguish between the present and the past. Think of a deep emotional wound as a virus in your computer. Even though you visited the website where your computer was infected months ago, the virus will continue to do its annoying thing as if it had been infected today. When your computer was infected, it does not matter. When very traumatic things happen to us, it is as if we play a CD with a scratch on it over and over. The subconscious mind responds to this traumatic event as a threat to its survival. Remember, to your subconscious mind, the traumatic event and the feelings it caused may as well be a real-life threat, like an angry bear. It is responding perfectly to *inappropriate information*.

Let's pretend for a minute that when you were ten years old, your abusive alcoholic father hit your mother. Unfortunately, you witnessed this event. Your subconscious mind responded to the intense fear the situation created as if your life were being threatened. It is still responding to this memory with the typical tools of survival. When you are scared, your blood pressure is elevated, you can't eat, and your muscles are tense and ready to fight. Only…there is no abusive father, simply the *memory* of him, churning destructively and unnoticed in the subconscious mind.

Your subconscious mind is responding to this memory as if it is a present danger. It cannot distinguish between present and past. Like the virus in your computer, it is ever-present, all the time, as if on a loop. To your subconscious mind, this is still happening *right now*. It is causing your digestive system to shut down, with your stomach in knots, your heart to pound with anxiety, and your blood pressure to be elevated.

Since you are not consciously *aware* of this memory very much alive in the subconscious state, wreaking havoc upon your body, these symptoms make no sense. They seem out of place and will usually eventually cause you to seek medical help. If you were to tell your doctor that you are scared and anxious all the time, you can't sleep, and your stomach hurts when you eat, he or she would most probably prescribe antianxiety medications, sleeping medications, or antidepressants, and refer you to a specialist for your digestive problems.

You are now chemically masking your physiological response to this buried memory. See the problem with this approach? The automatic (or autonomic) nervous system is so important that we will devote an entire chapter to it elsewhere. However, just know that there are upper cervical (neck) injuries that may cause your body to respond with the same fight-or-flight response, stuck in an endless loop.

Once called shell shock, PTSD is a serious condition that can develop after a person has experienced or witnessed a traumatic or terrifying event in which serious physical harm occurred or was threatened. PTSD is a lasting result of a traumatic experience that caused intense fear, helplessness, or horror, such as a sexual or physical assault, the unexpected death of a loved one, or an accident, war, or natural disaster. Patients who suffered sexual or physical abuse suffer from a high burden of stress upon their nervous systems and bodies, and are much more likely to develop chronic conditions such as CRPS.

Most people who experience a traumatic event will have reactions that may include shock, anger, nervousness, fear, and even guilt. These reactions are common, and for most people they go away over time. However, for a person with PTSD, these feelings continue and may even increase, becoming so strong that they keep the person from living a normal, happy life. People with PTSD have symptoms for longer than one month and cannot function as well as they did before the event occurred.

SO HOW DOES ONE AVOID...LIFE?

When I explain the effect emotional stress may have on their bodies to my patients, I almost always get this question: How does one avoid the bad things in life that seem to happen to all of us sooner or later? Remember, it is not *what* happens to us that make us physically sick; it is our *feelings* about these things that get our bodies stuck. So, are you supposed to stop feeling then? Just flip that handy-dandy "emotions off" switch in the back of your head? We are all human, after all. Although your emotions are 100 percent under your control, it is difficult to leave behind a lifetime of programming. When someone dies, we miss them. It makes us sad. When another driver is rude to us on the road, we get angry. How do we change the way we naturally respond to stress…with feeling? How do you friggin' neutralize negative feelings?

STEP 1: MAKE THE LINK
Understanding that *feelings* can make you physically sick is the first step. The founder of chiropractic, Dr. D. D. Palmer, used to say, "Be very careful who you rent the upstairs to." When you learn to watch your thoughts, based on the feelings you are feeling, you can begin to correct them. Awareness is the first step to healthier thinking. Most people just feel what they feel with abandon, with little thought of the consequence that those intense emotions may have upon their health. Every feeling has an effect upon your body; it can be a good effect or a bad effect.

STEP 2: QUIT ACTING LIKE AN OSTRICH
As adults, we deal with stress in various ways. One popular way is to simply "put it behind us," meaning, we bury it. However, as my good friend, Dr. David Pascal always says: "Burying stress is like burying toxic waste in your backyard. It always surfaces sooner or later." You have to acknowledge your feelings. As children, we are often taught that big boys and girls don't cry. It is implied that it is better to "suck it up," to keep our chins up, and to get over it. However, when you suppress an emotion, it will be expressed as a physical symptom. It will implode. Think of expressing your emotions as a pressure valve. It will keep your feelings from becoming toxic.

I am not necessarily advocating that you confront people who have upset you to their face; although this may be appropriate in some cases, it may also cause you too much anxiety. I, for one, despise confrontation. It reminds me of a funny joke here in the South: "I don't talk badly about people to their face. No, ma'am. My mamma raised me right. I do it *behind* their backs." I would rather drive needles through my skin with a hammer than confront people face to face. If you are like me and you would rather stuff your emotions down, I feel your pain. However, this is not a healthy way to live.

You have to learn to at least *own* your feelings. "When you said X to me, it made me feel Y. I understand that you did not necessarily mean to make me feel Y. These are just my feelings, which I am owning and taking responsibility for." Another great way of expressing your feelings is merely saying them out loud, even if no one else is around to hear you. I like to do this while I am driving or in the shower; that cuts down on the chances of other people thinking I have lost my marbles because I'm talking to myself. The mere act of saying something out loud counts as healthy expression. Think of it being said out loud with emotion as a release of negative energy from your body. Another solution is to write a letter or e-mail, even if you never send it. Many people find journaling helpful.

STEP 3: NEUTRALIZE THE ACID

Think back to your chemistry class in high school. How do you neutralize an acidic solution? You simply add an alkaline substance or solution. Think of your negative feelings as acid. It is corrosive and will eat away at you and your health unless neutralized. Whenever you find your thoughts about a memory to cause a negative emotion, mentally examine it until you can find some good in what happened.

Sometimes the only good you can find is the lesson you learned from that experience. Your lesson may be to not repeat that mistake, or to learn from the unpleasant feeling and vow to do better in the future, or maybe not to do unto others as has been done to you. Find at least one good thing in every unpleasant experience. It has to be there, by the law of polarity. Bad cannot exist without some good. The silver lining is there; just look for it.

My dad once had a patient whose husband was killed in front of her during a robbery. She asked him what good there was in that. His answer?

She was not killed. That may seem like a small thing, but it was a significant blessing amid that tragedy. While this is an extreme example, you get my drift. Find the nugget of good and acknowledge it. Of course, it is best to do this right away. Try not to spend months or years working through negative things that could be handled immediately. Even if it feels like you are just going through the motions, it is still incredibly effective. A little bit of positivity goes a very long way.

STEP 4: SELFISHLY FORGIVE OTHERS

> *Forgiveness is the fragrance that the violet sheds on the heel that has crushed it.*
>
> —Mark Twain

> *The weak can never forgive. Forgiveness is the attribute of the strong.*
>
> —Gandhi

> *Forgiveness is a gift you give yourself.*
>
> —Suzanne Somers

> *When you forgive, you in no way change the past—but you sure do change the future.*
>
> —Bernard Meltzer

The last step is forgiveness. People sometimes resist this step, since it feels as if they are condoning what was done to them by forgiving it. "It was not OK. I will not imply it was OK by forgiving them." Choose to look at it differently, however. Forgiveness is actually a very empowering action that will speed up your healing. It does not imply that you condone what was done to you. It simply means that you are choosing to let go. It is a very peaceful action, bringing you great return upon the investment of energy it takes to forgive. After all, what are you really letting go of? Anger. Grief. Resentment. Why would you choose to hang on to these negative emotions? Hatred is an acid that destroys its own container. Picture your hands opening and letting go of sharp, broken knife you were tightly holding on to, causing you pain. Just let go. Let it fall to the ground.

Forgiveness must be heartfelt, and more than just words spoken. While it takes a strong person to say "sorry," it takes an even stronger person to forgive. Forgiveness can be instant, or a gentle slow eroding of negative emotions as you keep focusing on any positives that came from the experience. Forgive the person, not the act. You will be healthier for it. You will be freer. Cut the ties that bind you with the most powerful sword in the world—forgiveness. Nothing binds you to a fellow human being more snugly than hatred.

STEP 5: FORGIVE YOURSELF

> *I have learned that the person I have to ask for forgiveness from the most is myself.*
>
> *You must love yourself.*
>
> *You have to forgive yourself, every day, whenever you remember a shortcoming, a flaw, you have to tell yourself, "That's just fine."*
>
> *You have to forgive yourself so much, until you don't even see those things anymore. Because that's what love is like.*
>
> —C. Joy Bell

I have noticed that my patients are hardest on themselves. We sometimes find it much easier to forgive others than ourselves. We somehow feel that if only we can beat ourselves up hard enough, we can go back in time and undo our bad decisions. Not marry that jerk. Not say hurtful things. Not take that dead-end job. Finish school. Never start smoking. Not have our hearts broken by people who should never have had the power to do so in the first place. Our lists of regrets are usually long and tough to admit. Yet we never let ourselves forget our own mistakes.

Please understand, we can only forgive others to the extent to which we can forgive ourselves. Do you understand how profound this is? The harder we are on ourselves, the harder we are on those around us and those we love. Be extra kind to yourself. Imagine yourself to be a student, moving through life's various classes. Sometimes we fail. Sometimes we fall down. A mistake is only a lesson waiting to be learned. Be as kind to you as you are to your most beloved friend or pet. Messing up is part of being human.

LYING IN WAIT: THE MAKINGS OF A MONSTER

> *Fate is like a strange, unpopular restaurant filled with odd little waiters who bring you things you never asked for and don't always like.*
>
> —Lemony Snicket

While stress (physical, emotional or chemical) cause all disease, it is my belief that CRPS is not the result of one single event or stress, but rather more like a complicated puzzle, made up of different parts. Stress only affects you adversely physically if you cannot adapt to it. People who suffer from CRPS became overwhelmed to the point that their bodies could not adjust or respond to stress, and CRPS was the unlucky result.

What then made your body so uniquely vulnerable to stress? While not every factor apply to every patient, a few general ones do apply in the majority of cases. Let us discuss those:

THE MTHFR GENE MUTATION (NO, IT'S NOT SHORT FOR A BAD WORD.)

You may or may not have ever heard of something called the MTHFR gene mutation. Inside your body, on a daily basis, countless metabolic and chemical cycles and processes take place every day right under your nose. Please stick with me, as this can get a little complicated even for those of us who love chemistry. You may not be aware of it, but your body is masterfully clever and complicated. MTHFR (Methylenetetrahydrofolate reductase) is an enzyme in the methyl cycle. During this cycle, a single molecule (known as the methyl donor) transfers a methyl group, consisting of three hydrogen atoms and one carbon atom to another molecule.

This causes the second molecule to become methylated, which is an essential process responsible for the production of something called glutathione. Glutathione is also known as the master detoxifier, and is known as the most powerful antioxidant inside our bodies. Glutathione is like the best maid in the world, cleaning up our toxic messes inside. It passes through each of our cells, dutifully collecting toxins and heavy metals in order to purge them from our body. Therefore, glutathione is responsible for the health and well-being of every single cell in your body.

What is the purpose of the methyl cycle? It is responsible for repairing damaged cells. When our cells are damaged by stress, free radicals or toxins, the methyl cycle inserts the new methyl group into the protein cell, where it goes to work to repair the damage. DNA cells are particularly dependent upon the methylation cycle to function properly, as it heavily influences the transformation of DNA information of the old DNA cells to the new DNA cells. Methylation is also responsible for neutralizing damaging homocysteine amino acids by turning them into methionine. The level of homocysteine in our body directly relates to our biological age. High levels will increase your chances of strokes, neurologic malfunction, heart disease, dementia, birth defects, high cholesterol, and many other conditions.⁹

MTHFR is a common genetic variant that causes this key enzyme to function at a lower than normal rate. In fact, a 2003 genetic study called the Human Genome Project was completed, surprisingly showing that a lot of people worldwide (some say as high as 60 percent of the population) are affected by this mutation. There are over fifty known variants of this gene, however, the two most common ones are called C677T (most commonly associated with heart attack and stroke) and A1298C (most commonly associated with a variety of chronic illnesses).

The MTHFR gene malfunction can be either heterozygous (meaning you have one affected gene and one normal gene, and that your enzyme activity will be about 60 percent normal) or homozygous (meaning you have two affected genes and that your enzyme activity could be as low as 10 percent). The worst-case scenario is 677T/1298C in which you are heterozygous to both anomalies. Many chronic illnesses have been linked to this unlucky anomaly.

Some of the symptoms associated with various forms of the MTHFR gene mutations are depression, anxiety, chronic pain, Parkinson's disease, CRPS, fibromyalgia, chronic fatigue, heart disease, elevated cholesterol, excessive clotting, glaucoma, frequent miscarriages, stillbirths, preeclampsia, birth defects in fetuses (such as spina bifida or cleft lip), autoimmune disorders, insomnia, and frequent headaches. Suffering from this mutation may put you at higher risk for addictions such as alcoholism and smoking.

In addition, this mutation will make it harder for your body to detoxify itself of various toxins. In fact, my CRPS patients often report that they simply do not tolerate medications or toxins as well as other people do, and that medications affect them very differently than most people. I commonly hear: "Doc, I am that one in a thousand. If something can go wrong, it will go wrong with my body. I always puzzle doctors." The same is true for alcohol. An inability to detoxify may also lead to thyroid disorders, menstrual disorders, kidney damage, liver damage, and cancer.

Although no formal study has ever been performed as of yet to link CRPS and the MTHFR gene mutation, it is my firm belief that such a link does exist. As mentioned previously, there is significant incidence of CRPS existing within families. In addition, fibromyalgia and CRPS share a significant overlap in both cause and presentation, if not exact symptoms. The link between the MTHFR gene mutation and fibromyalgia has been shown in various studies[10,11]

In addition, there is no doubt that CRPS involves an abnormally functioning nervous system. The nervous system has been shown to directly be affected by the MTHFR gene mutation.[12,13] While a lot of doctors can order the genetic test to screen for the MTHFR gene mutation, it is possible to also do a saliva test at home. One test currently available is at 23andme.com. This test will provide you with raw (and somewhat confusing) data. However, there are sites available that will interpret these results for you (e.g., geneticgenie.org or livewello.com).

Sometimes, routine blood testing will show abnormally high levels of folic acid in your body. This may also indicate that you suffer from the MTHFR mutation. The reason for this is that people who suffer from the C677T mutation do not process folic acid into methylfolate well. Supplemental and enriched folic acid foods (such as pastas) should be avoided as elevated folic acid levels have the potential to stimulate preexisting cancer cells. Active, methylated forms of folic acid are acceptable to take. Please see chapter 12 for more information.

It is important that you understand that I am not an advocate of being a victim of your genetic blueprint. While most of us are born with some genetic weaknesses, we are not slaves to these weaknesses. The information above should merely provide us with an action plan of fortifying and protecting our bodies with a specific goal or target in mind. I call this intelligent, proactive planning. As mentioned earlier, please familiarize yourself with the work of Dr. Bruce H. Lipton. His work teaches us that even though our DNA may contain genetic weaknesses, these weaknesses are much like locks, waiting for the right keys. The locks may be out of our control, but most of the keys as well as the unlocking process lie firmly within our control.

Just like a single cell, the character of our lives is determined not by our genes but by our responses to the environmental signals that propel life.

—Dr. Bruce Lipton

Next, as we explore the puzzle that is the making of CRPS, I will devote a few chapters to the central nervous system and its role in the development of CRPS.

5

The Playground Bully inside Your Nervous System

An old Cherokee is teaching his grandson about life. "A fight is going on inside me," he said to the boy.

"It is a terrible fight and it is between two wolves. One is evil—he is anger, envy, sorrow, regret, greed, arrogance, self-pity, guilt, resentment, inferiority, lies, false pride, superiority, and ego." He continued, "The other is good—he is joy, peace, love, hope, serenity, humility, kindness, benevolence, empathy, generosity, truth, compassion, and faith. The same fight is going on inside you—and inside every other person, too."

The grandson thought about it for a minute and then asked his grandfather, "Which wolf will win?"

The old Cherokee simply replied, "The one you feed."

—CHEROKEE LEGEND

Your hand opens and closes, opens and closes. If it were always a fist or always stretched open, you would be paralyzed. Your deepest presence is in every small *contracting and expanding, the two as beautifully balanced and coordinated as birds' wings.*

—Rumi

Never is harmony more important than inside the human body. Every biological process depends on a delicate balance. Actions that can be turned on, must also be able to be turned off. Things that are sped up should be able to be slowed down. When dealing with the central nervous system, this balance becomes particularly important. The reason for this is that the central nervous system is the foundation that runs every other cell, organ, and system inside of your body. For instance, it controls your sleep, immune system, hormones, healing, as well as pain levels. The central nervous system is composed of the brain and the spinal cord. I always tell my patients to think of the nervous system as the foundation of the body. If it is flawed or malfunctioning in any way, every other part of the body will be affected.

It is very important, when trying to understand how the human body works, to realize and appreciate how integral the central nervous system is to the body. When an embryo develops, the nervous system is the first to differentiate or form. It is the system that runs the entire body. It controls every single function or task that your body performs. If the brain is the captain, the spinal cord is the highway that carries the signals and commands to every cell and delivers feedback to this captain. It is the master control system. Every feeling of discomfort or pain involves the nervous system. In order for you to be healthy, this system has to be healthy.

THE AUTONOMIC NERVOUS SYSTEM

In this chapter, we take a closer look at the autonomic (or automatic) nervous system. While I don't need you to become an expert on neurology (who has the time?), I do want to make sure that you have a good basic understanding of how this system works and what it controls (everything!) so that many of the mysterious neurological symptoms associated with CRPS will make sense. When you understand how something started going haywire in the first place, you can begin the process of fixing it.

Typically, our current health-care system consists of managing symptoms. This can be done in many different ways. Nerve signals of pain and discomfort are seen as a bothersome and unwanted symptom and may be numbed or interrupted. Nerves may be removed. Organs will also often be removed. If a part hurts, it must be silenced, numbed, or taken out. Today, this way of thinking has become normal for most of us.

What I am about to say may sound extreme, but I stand by it. Unless the body is in an extreme emergency situation where immediate action is needed to prevent permanent damage, organ loss, or death, medical management of symptoms rarely contributes to longevity or improved health, and most often may actually take away from the patient's overall quality of life. Please note that under some circumstances, such as Parkinson's, symptom management is very understandable and appropriate. However, generally speaking, symptom management should preferably be exercised only for limited periods of time.

All that being said, it's understandable *why* CRPS sufferers desperately reach for relief in the form of a pill, spinal cord stimulator, or infusion. Anything, *anything* to put out the fire. It is impossible to function in everyday life while in excruciating pain. However, such management of pain should never be confused with a healing process or improved health. Please note that I do not judge anyone who suffers from CRPS who needs pain relief. My hope is simply for you to find the answers that will make it possible for you to live without daily pain medication.

Let's take a closer look at the autonomic nervous system and how it causes some of the most common symptoms associated with CRPS.

The autonomic nervous system is a control system within your peripheral and sensory nervous system that influences the function of internal organs. This system acts largely automatically without any conscious input from you, and regulates bodily functions such as digestion, sexual arousal, respiration, heart rate, blood pressure, and urination, to name a few. Certain reflex actions such as sneezing, coughing, and vomiting are also controlled by the autonomic nervous system. Within the brain, the autonomic nervous system is controlled by the hypothalamus. The hypothalamus is located just above the brain stem within the brain.

This system is divided into the sympathetic and parasympathetic nervous system. The sympathetic nervous system is largely responsible for speeding up functions in the body, and is known as the "fight or flight" system. The parasympathetic nervous system is considered the "rest and digest" or "feed and breed" nervous system, and mostly is responsible for slowing functions down inside the body. Think of the sympathetic nervous system as the gas pedal in your car, and of the parasympathetic nervous system as the brake.

PEDAL TO THE MEDAL: THE ONE THING EVERY SINGLE CRPS PATIENT'S NERVOUS SYSTEM HAS IN COMMON

What if your body was an airplane and your pilot drunk? The autonomic nervous system (sometimes known as the automatic or involuntary nervous system) is incredibly important to your health, as this system is the master control system that runs every single function in your body. Most of these functions require no conscious thought from you. You don't have to remember to breathe, for example. When you are sitting in an airplane, you don't have to know exactly what the pilot is doing up there in the cabin. You just trust that he is doing his job and will keep the plane in the air and eventually land it safely. In the case of most CRPS sufferers, the pilot is unfortunately up to all sorts of monkey business, and usually has his hand frozen in the full-throttle position.

The sympathetic and parasympathetic nervous systems have exactly opposite effects on the functions of the body. They essentially work in opposition to each other, but in a way that complements each other. As I said earlier, think of your sympathetic nervous system as the gas pedal, and the parasympathetic nervous system as the brake pedal. The balance between the two is *crucial* for the perfect function of every cell in your body. While they are both crucial to the car, they cannot be stepped on at the same time.

In every single CRPS patient, the sympathetic nervous system has its pedal to the metal, all the time. This may be the case years before you ever develop CRPS, or your nervous system may be injured resulting in this imbalance when you suffer from the traumatic injury that triggered your CRPS. As many CRPS sufferers unfortunately find out firsthand, this is bad news for your health. The golden rule of the autonomic nervous system is that if one system is up, the other system must be down.

THE SYMPATHETIC NERVOUS SYSTEM: "FIGHT OR FLIGHT"

This system was designed to help your body fight to stay alive when your survival is being threatened. Think of a caveman in hand-to-paw combat with a saber-toothed tiger. This portion of your nervous system responds very quickly (think zero to ninety in a few seconds), since one usually doesn't have time to calmly ponder one's response to a life-threatening situation. When your life is being threatened and your body gets ready to fight in order to ensure its survival, every small bit of energy spent is carefully considered. Nothing is wasted. Energy will be rerouted away from systems that do not concern themselves with short-term survival, to where it can be used more readily to fight an immediate threat. For example, blood will flow away from the digestive tract and skin in order to be rationed out to the lungs and muscles. It is more important under those circumstances to be able to fight using your muscles, and to breathe hard and fast, as your body needs oxygen.

Speaking of oxygen, the bronchioles (small air passages) in the lungs will open up, which allows for more oxygen into the blood. At the same time the heart will beat faster. Another physiological change in the body is that the pupils will dilate, allowing more light to enter the eyes. The adrenal glands on top of the kidneys will pump adrenalin in case you need extra motivation besides fear to fight. It will also make all the sphincters (think of pressure valves) in the body, like the urinary sphincter, contract and close tight.

So why does this affect you? There probably isn't the equivalent of a saber-toothed tiger chasing you every day. Your brain cannot distinguish fear and stress from *actual* life-threatening situations. Additionally, as mentioned earlier in this book when we discussed emotional stress, a very old traumatic event can run in a continuous "loop" in the subconscious mind. The brain cannot distinguish between this old memory and present danger. The old memory almost acts like a computer virus, messing with the software in your nervous system. Your brain does not know that it *isn't happening anymore.*

When a person suffers an emotionally traumatic event or a neck injury following, for example, a fall or car accident affecting the brain stem directly or indirectly, the sympathetic nervous system will become overexcited, affecting the whole body.[14–16] This will cause your sympathetic nervous system, or fight-or-flight response, to be stuck in the "on" position day in and day out—and if your sympathetic nervous system is stuck all the time, your parasympathetic nervous system is turned off. Instead of these two systems working in perfect harmony, the sympathetic nervous system turns into the schoolyard bully, or the puppet master, pulling your body's strings and directing it on a disastrous course every second of the day. This will create the perfect conditions inside your body that put you at risk to develop CRPS and other autonomic dysfunction or WAD (whiplash-associated dysfunctions). I will discuss each symptom in detail, after we explain how the parasympathetic nervous system works.

THE PARASYMPATHETIC NERVOUS SYSTEM: "REST AND DIGEST" OR "FEED AND BREED"

Think of your parasympathetic nervous system as the system that calms you down, helps you to rest and sleep, helps to facilitate healing in the body, and deals with sexual arousal. It functions to counter the sympathetic system. After a crisis or danger has passed, this system helps to calm the body. Your heart and breathing rates slow, your digestion resumes, your pupils contract, and you stop sweating.

This system will also cause the increase of blood flow to your GI tract following a meal to allow digestion. It stimulates the movements of your intestines (called *peristalsis*) that move food through your intestines. It will constrict the pupil of the eye, cause you to salivate when appropriate, and is responsible for getting you in the mood for sex. This system, if activated, will activate your immune system, cause increased circulation to the skin and extremities, and help to release your "feel-good" hormones, called endorphins. It will also decrease temperature. It is the main control system that promotes healing. This system is usually underactive, suppressed, or turned off in those who suffer from CRPS. No wonder you are not in the mood for getting frisky!

THE VAGUS NERVE: YOUR SEVERED LIFELINE

If you suffer from CRPS, you should familiarize yourself with the vagus nerve, as it is a major player in building the puzzle that forms CRPS. The vagus nerve is the single most important nerve inside the human body outside of the spinal cord. It is one of twelve pairs of cranial nerves. These nerves emerge directly from the brain and brain stem, as opposed to spinal nerves that emerge from the sides of the spinal cord. Each cranial nerve is paired and is present on both sides. The cranial nerves provide motor and sensory information mainly to the structures of the head and neck (think sensations like smell, taste, hearing, or vision, for example.) These nerves are numbered by roman numerals. The vagus nerve is the tenth nerve (CN X), and it is the longest cranial nerve.

Please stick with me here, as I realize that some of you may be bored by the anatomy of the nervous system. I promise that this nerve matters greatly in the development (and therefore also the healing) of the neurological symptoms of CRPS.

The vagus nerve (meaning "wandering nerve") has multiple branches that diverge from two thick stems rooted in the cerebellum and brain stem that wander to the lowest viscera of your abdomen also connecting to your heart and most major organs along the way, such as the lungs. The vagus nerve supplies motor parasympathetic fibers to *all* the organs except the adrenal glands, from the neck down to the transverse colon. The vagus nerve is responsible for many different tasks, including (but not limited to): heart rate, digestion, sweating, speech, coughing, fainting, and vomiting, to name but a few. Remember, people who suffer from CRPS also suffer from sympathetic dominance (the schoolyard bully), causing the parasympathetic nervous system to be suppressed and to shut down. This means that people who suffer from CRPS also suffer, by definition, from an underactive vagus nerve.

Just to recap: the parasympathetic nervous system is responsible (in general) for slowing and calming things down, as well as healing and sleep. The vagus nerve forms an electric circuit that links our heart, digestive tract, and lungs to the brain. Let's look at how this nerve affects specific organs just a bit closer.

YOUR ACHY BREAKY HEART

In a normal heart, the resting heart rate is controlled by the parasympathetic nervous system. It has been shown that the resting heart rate (meaning your heart rate when you aren't engaged in physical activity) is a measure of your vagus nerve function and predicts mortality. The vagus nerve also controls inflammation in the body. This topic is so important that we will later devote an entire chapter to it. For now, I did want to mention, however, that vagus-nerve suppression will lead to inflammation of the tissue of the heart, causing tissue injury, preventing remodeling of cells, and leading to cell death. Vagus-nerve stimulation, in turn, will prevent tissue injury and cell death in the heart.[17,18]

The higher the vagus nerve activity is, the greater the increase in the parasympathetic component of heart rate variability is, the slower your heart rate is, and the better the outcome is. In people who suffer from heart failure, heart rate is less regulated by parasympathetic activation. There is a clear relationship between increased heart rate and adverse outcomes, such as heart failure.

CRPS patients are particularly vulnerable to cardiac disease and malfunction. While no specific study has been performed to link the incidence of cardiac disease and CRPS, it is my belief that such a link does exist.

JUST BREATHE: HOW THE VAGUS NERVE AFFECTS YOUR LUNGS

The vagus nerve is one of the key players that help you to breathe and keep your lungs healthy. When the lung expands during normal breathing, the vagus nerve sends a message to the brain that causes the bronchi to constrict. We cannot survive without oxygen for more than five minutes. Therefore, breathing is essential not only to our health, but to our very survival. There is an undeniable link between an overactive immune system, inflammation, and breathing disorders such as asthma, COPD (Chronic Obstructive Pulmonary Disease) and sleep apnea.[19] Sleep apnea is actually very common among people who suffer from fibromyalgia and CRPS. When you are not breathing correctly, it will also affect your sleep at night, which in turn affects healing. Healing happens much more effectively during deep, quality REM sleep than your waking hours.

In addition, proper breathing is very vital to maintain the health of your brain and central nervous system. During relaxed abdominal breathing, your brainwaves will also show a pattern of relaxation. The vagus nerve uses a neurotransmitter called acetylcholine that communicates with the diaphragm which is essential for breathing.

It is interesting that not only does the vagus nerve help to regulate your breathing, but you can activate the vagus nerve in return by using specific breathing, namely slow, deep breaths, breathing from the abdomen, and exhaling longer than you inhale. When we think of breathing, we tend to focus on oxygen only. The truth is that breathing serves other functions as well. Exhaling carbon dioxide is actually a powerful detoxification pathway in the body. We literally breathe out our waste (hence morning breath). When our lungs are not doing so effectively, we overburden our other detoxification pathways, such as the kidneys and liver.

When the lungs expand and contract it has an effect on the body that is almost like a pumping action, much like the heart, but bigger. It is responsible for tissue repair, lymphatic drainage of waste products, activation of the immune system, and dilation of blood vessels that is crucial for healing, to name but a few.

GUT FEELINGS ARE ACTUALLY REAL: HOW THE VAGUS NERVE CONNECTS WITH YOUR EMOTIONS

The vagus nerve is constantly sending real-time sensory information about the body's organs to your brain via nerves called afferent nerves, meaning, leading into the brain. Efferent nerves, in turn, lead out of the brain. About 90 percent of the nerve fibers in the vagus nerve are dedicated to communicating the state of your organs to your brain every nanosecond.

Gut instincts are not imaginary, but are actual emotional signals transferred to your brain via the vagus nerve. Signals from the vagus nerve traveling from your gut to your brain have been linked to changes in your mood and emotions such as fear and anxiety. Underlying these gut feelings is a little-known network of neurons lining our guts like tiny fingers that is so sophisticated that some call it our second brain. These nerves are filled with neurotransmitters and does much more than merely controlling digestion. This second brain (called the enteric nervous system) in our insides, together with the brain in our heads, help to determine our emotional state and also play a key role in certain diseases throughout the body.

Although its influence is far-reaching, the second brain is not the seat of any conscious thoughts or decision-making. The enteric nervous system contains about a hundred million neurons, more than in either the spinal cord or the peripheral nervous system put together. It consists of sheaths of interconnected neurons embedded in the walls of the long tube of our gut, which measures about twenty-nine feet from the esophagus to the anus. The enteric nervous system enables our brain to be in touch with the inner world of our gut, although it is not capable of rational thought, such as putting together a shopping list.

A big part of our emotions is influenced by the nerves in our gut. Butterflies in the stomach, which is a typical stress response, is one example of this. The enteric nervous system uses more than thirty neurotransmitters, just like the brain, and in fact about 95 percent of the body's serotonin is produced in the gut. Depression has been shown to be directly linked to abnormalities in the gut, affecting serotonin levels.[20]

JEEPERS CREEPERS: HOW UNHEALTHY GUT BACTERIA CONTROL YOU AND YOUR HABITS

Inside our gut live millions of bacteria, some good, and some bad, together weighing about as much as our brain. When we are healthy, the good bacteria far outweighs the bad. The vagus nerve can actually alert our brain if this balance is tipped toward the unhealthy bacteria, if it is functioning correctly. If we are unhealthy, the bad can overcome the good in numbers, leading to dire consequences. Much like people, different bacteria need different foods in order to thrive. Some prefer fats, and some prefer sugar. Some even recognize and are repulsed by the supplements that may kill or harm it. While it is unclear exactly how this occurs, it has been shown that this diverse community of bacteria, collectively known as the gut microbiome, may influence our decisions by releasing signaling molecules into our gut. It is almost as if we have millions of little aliens in our guts.

Because the gut is linked to the immune system, the endocrine system and the nervous system, those signals could influence our physiologic and behavioral responses as well as our choices of, for example, the food we eat.[21] In other words, the bugs in our gut manipulate us to pick the foods that they prefer. They will also release unpleasant chemicals in our blood when we take a supplement or eat foods that can kill them. This is why the supplements or foods that your body sometimes needs the most will physically repulse you. Microbes will also affect our mood and emotional state. Microbes have the capacity to manipulate behavior and mood through altering the neural signals in the vagus nerve, producing toxins to make us feel bad, and releasing chemical rewards to make us feel good.

Fortunately, you are still in control of our own body, and you can evict these toxic little unwanted squatters. How? You can actually use food to kill off bad bugs in our gut, and do so fast. As a matter of fact, as soon as you change your eating habits, changes can be measured within as early as twenty-four hours. For this reason, we will cover diet and supplementation in more detail later in this book.

LEAKY GUT AND ALLERGIES

Patients who suffer from intestinal disorders, such as a leaky gut, will often develop allergies.[22] What exactly is a leaky gut? This should be of interest to you, as the majority of CRPS patients suffer from it. Normally, the intestinal lining forms a barrier between all the stuff we eat and our blood. This protects our bodies and also filters needed nutrients from unwanted ones. The small intestine is designed to allow very small particles of digested nutrients to pass through its wall and into the bloodstream, where it is distributed throughout the body as needed.

Due to a variety of causes, the intestinal wall can become more permeable or "leaky" and allow larger, half-digested food particles or toxins and waste to pass through, causing what is known as leaky gut syndrome. The cause of this may be decreased nervous system communication to the gut, resulting in "bad housekeeping" and damage to the gut, which is most often the case in CRPS. Other possible causes may be chronic inflammation, using the birth control pill, chronic emotional stress, food sensitivities, a sluggish liver, damage from taking large amounts of nonsteroidal anti-inflammatory drugs (NSAIDS), medications, radiation or certain antibiotics, excessive and long-term alcohol, caffeine or tobacco use, too much sugar, heavy-metal toxicity, candida overgrowth, or decreased immunity.

When these particles enter the bloodstream, the immune system recognizes them as foreign invaders and attempts to fight them off. Over a long period of time, this will cause your immune system to malfunction and may result in autoimmune conditions and allergies. The first step in treating leaky gut syndrome and other GI problems in a CRPS patient should be restoring proper nervous system communication to the GI system, as discussed elsewhere in this book.

WHEN EATING BECOMES TORTURE: THE VAGUS NERVE AND YOUR DIGESTIVE SYSTEM

One of the symptoms that is pretty universal in all CRPS patients, besides pain, is digestive issues. These issues will be varied, depending upon the patient and how long they have been sick. In its mild first stages, patients usually suffer from indigestion, heartburn, constipation or diarrhea, and bloating. As it progresses, patients may suffer from food allergies, leaky gut syndrome, Crohn's disease, and chronic inflammation of the GI tract. In its most severe form, patients will suffer from gastroparesis, or weakness (paralysis) of the muscles of the stomach.

The vagus nerve helps manage many complicated processes in your digestive tract, including signaling the muscles in your stomach to contract and push food into the small intestine. A malfunctioning vagus nerve can't send signals to your stomach muscles. This results in poor digestion of the food in your stomach, and the slowing down of the emptying of your stomach. Patients who suffer from this condition will have a very difficult time ingesting anything other than liquids. This condition results in nausea, vomiting, and severe abdominal pain. CRPS patients suffering from GI problems are usually treated like patients with two separate conditions, rather than a patient with a central nervous system malfunction resulting in both conditions. The distinction here is an important one, as one treatment approach works, and the other doesn't.

Medical treatment of GI problems usually involves prescribing medication(s) to manage symptoms (for instance to force the bowels to function more regularly) and under very extreme circumstances, surgery to remove malfunctioning parts. Diet is rarely addressed, and even when it is addressed, it is done so poorly. Managing symptoms without addressing the root cause is like putting a wet towel over a fire alarm while the house is burning down. This approach is not only ineffective, it is actually harmful. In order to tackle this problem logically, you must first understand *why* the GI system started malfunctioning in the first place.

SLEEP, A DISTANT MEMORY

This quote reminds me of CRPS patients: "Remember when you woke up all refreshed after going to bed early and drifting off to sleep easily? Me either." Besides the constant pain, sleeping problems are probably one of the most annoying and life-robbing symptoms CRPS patients suffer from.

Sleeping serves a very important function. While you are sleeping, your nervous system has much more energy available for healing. There are many reasons for this. During this time, you are not thinking. Thinking invariably evokes emotions, which requires some of your available energy to be spent. Your senses are, for the most part, shut down. You are not hearing, seeing, or smelling. You are not using your large muscle groups to move around. All the energy normally used on these functions can now be redirected and used to assist your body in the healing process. However, if you are sleep-deprived, your body is missing out on this golden opportunity. It is estimated that your body heals about three times faster while asleep. It is a cruel twist of fate that the patients who need this most are the very patients who can't sleep.

Sleep problems with CRPS include insomnia or difficulty falling asleep as well as waking up frequently. An even more common problem is frequently waking up even though you don't remember doing so the next day, which interrupts your "deep" sleep. Also, other sleep disorders, such as restless leg syndrome and sleep apnea, may be associated with CRPS. Add to this the constant, tearing pain, which prevents deep restful sleep in itself.

My patients suffering from CRPS tell me that they wake up day after day feeling exhausted with no energy. Usually, people who suffer from CRPS feel more tired in the morning and many go back to sleep during the day to attempt to alleviate their fatigue. Also, it's common for people with CRPS to have great difficulty focusing during the day, a symptom made worse by the fibro fog a lot of them already suffer from. While brain fog is often attributed to sleep deprivation, it is my belief that brain fog is not caused by insomnia, but rather made worse by it. The involvement of the cranial nerves, together with severe inflammation affecting the brain, are much likelier culprits.

While almost every CRPS patient under allopathic care is prescribed some form of sleep medication, these medications only treat the symptom of sleeplessness, and often poorly. If you want to restore deep sleep, it is crucial that the malfunctioning autonomic nervous system be balanced. Remember, your parasympathetic nervous system is not working correctly, and the parasympathetic nervous system controls your rest. To make matters worse, the less you sleep, the more severe your pain, which, in turn, leads to even poorer sleep.

AVOID BLUE LIGHTS (AND WE AREN'T TALKING ABOUT THE POLICE.)

The color, determined by the wavelength, of the light we see sets our biological clocks, also known as circadian rhythms. In the natural environment, in caveman (and woman) days, this worked out pretty well. During the day, we see all the visible wavelengths provided by the sun—blue, violet, green, yellow, orange, and red light. This light communicates to our bodies that it's daytime, time to shake a tail feather and be active. During this time, secretion of your "sleepy hormone," melatonin, is decreased.

At night, melatonin is not affected by traditionally visible light, which consists of longer wavelengths—the yellows, oranges, and reds that we create through campfires or candles. Melatonin is released by your body, like the sandman dishing out dream sand. This allows us to get sleepy right when we are supposed to, together with a large part of the animal kingdom. Lullaby and goodnight.

However, we don't use candles and fire at night anymore. We stare at our TV screens, which emanate blue light. We work on our laptops (as I am doing now)—more blue light. We use our iPhones and other smartphones—you guessed it, blue light. If we wake up in the middle of the night, we can't resist checking our e-mail or our Facebook accounts (maybe somebody else is awake and liked our clever post about how annoying flossing is!)

Ditto iPads and e-readers. (If you are reading this at night on one of those devices, you are suppressing your melatonin as we speak. Finish this paragraph and step away from the blue light.) Our bodies associate blue light with daytime. Blue light wakes up your brain, resets your body clock, and suppresses melatonin all at the same time. The closer your face is to the device, the worse the problem.

If you own an iPad, its blue light emissions can be reduced by adjusting the brightness and switching to White on Black mode at night through the "settings" feature. If not, you can now purchase blue light filters for your computer, e-reader, iPad, or smartphone. (Just Google "blue light filters.")

EXHAUSTION

While most people who suffer from CRPS attribute their daily exhaustion to pain, sleeplessness or poor quality sleep, it is usually not the only reason they feel exhausted every day. Adrenal fatigue is also a likely culprit.

Each smaller than a walnut, your two adrenal glands sit on top of your kidneys. These relatively small hormone-producing glands are powerhouses, manufacturing and secreting almost fifty different hormones including adrenalin, cortisol (stress hormone that affects things like fat storage, blood sugar, and blood pressure), estrogen, testosterone, and aldosterone (regulating salt and water levels in the body). They significantly affect the function of every organ and tissue down to every cell in your body.

When these glands are not working properly, your immune system as well as your energy level will be affected. Even your mood may be affected, causing you to see the world through a rather gray lens. When these glands are malfunctioning, your health may also be severely compromised, and you will live below your optimal potential. The adrenal glands are responsible for ensuring that your body's reactions to stress are appropriate to optimize survival, without harming the body in return. For example, the adrenal glands are responsible for secreting protective hormones to help minimize allergic reactions such as swelling.

Adrenal fatigue is a syndrome where these glands malfunction or become fatigued due to working harder and longer than they were designed to do. This may happen after chronic or acute infections, after periods of intense stress such as losing a loved one, or during prolonged stress such as having a stressful job. It may also be caused by malfunctioning of the autonomic nervous system (as is the case in patients who suffer from CRPS). When the brain is "stuck" on sympathetic (fight-or-flight) overdrive, it is like your body is functioning while you are flooring the gas pedal 24/7. In response, these glands are frantically responding to this unseen stressful situation, for example, by pumping out adrenalin. Eventually, they become exhausted, leading to adrenal fatigue.

So, why don't allopathic doctors generally diagnose adrenal fatigue? Doctors are only taught to look for extreme adrenal malfunction in medical school. This includes Cushing's syndrome, which stems from too much cortisol production, or Addison's disease, which occurs when the adrenal glands don't produce enough cortisol. Traditionally, allopathic physicians check adrenal function by testing ACTH levels, using a bell curve to recognize abnormal levels. The ACTH test (also called the cosyntropin test, tetracosactide test, or Synacthen test) is a test usually ordered and interpreted by endocrinologists to assess the functioning of the adrenal glands, by measuring their stress response to adrenocorticotropic (ACTH) hormone.

The problem with this test is that when it is interpreted, only the top and bottom 2 percent of the curve are considered abnormal, yet symptoms of adrenal malfunction occur after 15 percent of the mean on both sides of the curve. In other words, your adrenal glands can be functioning 20 percent below the mean and the rest of your body experiencing all the symptoms of adrenal fatigue, yet most mainstream physicians won't diagnose you with an adrenal problem.

SIGNS OF ADRENAL FATIGUE

- Chronic fatigue and exhaustion (not relieved by sleep), usually worse in the morning and slightly better after 6:00 p.m.

- Decreased sex drive
- Inability to lose weight
- Tendency to carry excess weight in the belly area
- Recurrent infections and decreased immune system
- Lung problems such as bronchitis and asthma
- Allergies
- Sudden dizziness when you stand up from a lying or sitting position
- Muscle aches and weakness
- Depression, sadness, and a general gloomy outlook on life
- Salt or sugar cravings
- Swelling
- Excessive urination
- Hemorrhoids
- Feeling overwhelmed by even minor stress
- Struggling to get through the day
- Symptoms of hypoglycemia (shakiness, dizziness, sweating)

Please note that this list is not meant to replace a professional diagnosis, and that it is not all-inclusive.

HOW TO GET TESTED FOR ADRENAL FATIGUE AT HOME

In his book *Adrenal Fatigue*, which I highly recommend, James L. Wilson, DC, ND, PhD, describes three methods you may use at home to help determine high probability of adrenal fatigue.

1) **The Iris Contraction Test**

    For this test, you will need a mirror, a stopwatch (or a watch with a second hand), and a darkened room.

    In a darkened room, sit in a chair in front of a mirror. Holding the flashlight at the side of your head, shine it across one eye (not into the eye). Watch what happens to your eye in the mirror. The pupil should immediately contract when exposed to the light, and stay contracted. If you suffer from adrenal fatigue, however, the pupil won't be able to hold its contraction and will dilate. This dilation will take place within two minutes and last for about thirty to forty-five seconds before it contracts again. Time how long the dilation lasts and record it along with the date. Retest monthly as it serves as an indicator of recovery.

2) **The Blood Pressure Test** (aka Ragland's test)
In order to perform this test, you will need a blood pressure cuff (the type that does not require a stethoscope).

Make sure you are well hydrated before doing this test; otherwise it will give you a false positive. Lie down quietly for about ten minutes, and then take your blood pressure while still lying down. Then stand up and measure your blood pressure immediately upon standing. Normally blood pressure will rise ten to twenty mmHg from standing up. If your blood pressure drops, you likely have adrenal fatigue. The more severe the drop is, the more severe the adrenal fatigue you are suffering from.

3) **Sergeant's White Line**
This is the simplest of the home tests. With the capped end of a ballpoint pen, lightly stroke the skin on your abdomen, making a mark about six inches long. Within a few seconds, a line should appear. In a normal reaction, the mark is initially white, but reddens within a few seconds. If you have adrenal fatigue, the line will stay white for about two minutes and will also widen. Please note that if positive, this is an absolute confirmation. However, this sign is only present in 40 percent of people with adrenal fatigue.

ANOTHER TEST I RECOMMEND: SALIVA TESTING

Cortisol output by your adrenal glands is one of the most reliable indicators of your adrenal function and how well your body is dealing with stress. According to adrenalfatigue.org, the cortisol/DHEAS saliva test measures the levels of the stress hormones DHEAS and cortisol in your saliva, and provides an evaluation of how these levels differ throughout the day.

(For more about this test, go to www.adrenalfatigue.org.) Another condition that shares close symptoms with adrenal fatigue is an underactive thyroid gland, or hypothyroidism.

UNDERACTIVE THYROID (OR WHY LOOKING AT A COOKIE MAKES YOU GAIN TWO POUNDS)

The thyroid gland is located in the front of the neck, just below the Adam's apple. The two-inch gland consists of two lobes and is one of the largest endocrine glands in our bodies.

The function of the thyroid gland is to take iodine, found in many foods, such as seaweed, and convert it into thyroid hormones triiodothyronine (T3) and thyroxine (T4). Thyroid cells are the only cells in the body that can absorb iodine. These cells combine iodine and the amino acid tyrosine to make T3 and T4. T3 and T4 are then released into the bloodstream (the great transportation system) and are circulated throughout the body, where they control your metabolism. Metabolism is the conversion of oxygen and calories into energy. This is why the thyroid is known as the fat-burning gland. Every cell in the body depends upon thyroid hormones for regulation of its metabolism. In addition, the thyroid gland plays an important role in regulating your body's calcium levels.

The thyroid gland, in turn, is controlled by the hypothalamus (a small area above the brain stem) and the pituitary gland (a small gland the size of a peanut, lying beneath the hypothalamus). The hypothalamus helps to coordinate the nervous and endocrine systems. It passes signals to the pituitary gland, which in turn helps to regulate growth, maturation, and metabolism.

When the body is in fight-or-flight mode, or the autonomic nervous system is activated, the hypothalamus sends signals to the pituitary to secrete several hormones. Adrenocorticotropic hormone acts on the adrenal gland to secrete cortisol, and TSH (thyroid-stimulating hormone) acts on the thyroid gland to secrete thyroid hormones.

REMEMBER: THE NERVOUS SYSTEM OF A CRPS SUFFERER IS OFTEN STUCK IN SYMPATHETIC OVERDRIVE.

The result of this response is that the thyroid gland of the patient who suffers from CRPS often stops working correctly. In addition, the patient's immune system is often malfunctioning, leading to autoimmune conditions where the body attacks the thyroid gland.

SIGNS OF A THYROID THAT ISN'T WORKING

- Fatigue
- Infertility
- Increased sensitivity to cold or heat
- Coarse, dry, scaly, or thick skin
- Constipation
- Difficulty concentrating
- Unexplained weight gain
- Carpal tunnel syndrome
- Puffiness and swelling around the eyes and face
- Hoarseness
- Muscle weakness
- Elevated blood cholesterol level
- Muscle aches, tenderness, and stiffness
- Pain, stiffness, or swelling in your joints
- Heavier than normal or irregular menstrual periods
- Thinning hair
- Slowed heart rate
- Depression
- Impaired memory
- Frequent urination
- Impotence
- Brittle nails

- Poor exercise tolerance
- Panic attacks
- Anxiety

HOW TO GET TESTED FOR A SLUGGISH THYROID? HAVE BOTH T3 AND T4 TESTED

It is very common for CRPS patients to exhibit many of the symptoms listed above, and test negative for hypothyroidism (sluggish thyroid) when their blood is tested by their allopathic doctor. It doesn't seem to matter if you are exhibiting all of the classic signs of hypothyroidism; if the test indicates that your thyroid is normal, your doctor will typically agree with it. Doctors can be stubborn and old-fashioned like that. It is up to you, the patient (and the person who cares about your body and health the most), to inform yourself about your symptoms, the tests available to you, the tests needed in your case, and the reasons you ought to have these tests.

TSH: THE OLD GUARD'S WAY

The TSH (thyroid-stimulating hormone) has become the "gold standard" of thyroid function. When most doctors do a thyroid test, they measure your TSH and decide, based on the test result, whether you have a thyroid problem or not. The typical reference ranges (the numbers below and above which the tests are considered abnormal) are too broad to catch minor fluctuations of the thyroid that may still be symptomatic. Also, these tests are, of course, generalized and do not consider individual differences in physiology.

Even if doctors go a step further, beyond just testing the TSH, and look at your free T4, they will typically not look at your T3 levels. This way, there is no way of knowing if your body is properly converting the T4 it makes into T3. (T4 is the inactive form of thyroid hormone. It must be converted to T3 before the body can use it). This conversion can be decreased because of inflammation or high cortisol levels. Often, regardless of your TSH testing normal, your T3 will be low, resulting in symptoms.

The TSH does not reflect the whole body, but only the function of your brain tissue. According to an expert in the treatment of the thyroid gland, David M. Derry, MD, PhD, thyroid metabolism is controlled locally in the tissue by each organ in very individual and distinct ways. The brain has one mechanism for controlling the amount of thyroid available to the brain, but it is different from that used for other tissues such as the liver. There are many mechanisms by which each tissue controls the amount of thyroid hormone it needs. When TSH is tested, that only reflects thyroid metabolism in *one* of your organs—the brain.

Additionally, monitoring only the TSH levels of someone undergoing treatment for a sluggish thyroid is also going to lead to undertreating the patient. The pituitary cells are the most sensitive cells in the body when it comes to circulating thyroid hormone. Therefore, if your doctor treats hypothyroidism by following the TSH and trying to make it normal, the pituitary cells are happy, but the rest of the body may not be getting nearly the amount it needs. (For more information, please research the work of Dr. Derry.)

THYROID ANTIBODY TEST

If you suffer from CRPS, you should ask your doctor to include the thyroid antibodies tests to detect autoimmune disease, due to the fact that the immune system of a CRPS patient is usually not functioning optimally and autoimmune conditions in this group are common.

REVERSE T3 (AKA TRIIODOTHYRONINE)

When your thyroid is healthy, it produces several hormones. These include T1, T2, T3, T4, and RT3 (reverse T3). T4 is a storage hormone that converts into a more active hormone, T3, as needed. Sometimes, the body just needs to get rid of excess T4, and it then converts T4 into RT3. This is mostly done by the liver. Roughly 40 percent of T4 is converted into T3 and 20 percent into RT3. However, if your body is stressed, which results in high cortisol and low adrenals, the conversion into RT3 is sped up to convert about 50 percent of T4 into RT3. This results in low T3 levels, which, as you probably can guess, are not good. Therefore, we suggest that you also get tested for RT3 (reverse T3), especially if your other thyroid tests are inconclusive.

THE TEMPERATURE TEST

It is well known that a slow metabolism is a very common sign of sluggish thyroid glands. Your metabolism will directly affect your body temperature. Therefore, taking your temperature may be an important clue if you suspect that your thyroid gland is underactive. However, please note that this test is somewhat controversial in its accuracy and should not be used as a stand-alone diagnostic tool.

The temperature of an adult with a healthy thyroid and a healthy metabolism is (on average) 37.0 degrees Celsius or 98.6 degrees Fahrenheit. The best time to measure this is around 3:00 p.m. If you take your midafternoon temp and find it in the low 98s or even in the 97s, you have been given a strong clue that you may have an underactive thyroid.

Another good time to take your temperature is in the morning before you get out of bed. A normal morning basal temp should be between 97.8 and 98.2. If it's higher, you may be hyperthyroid, and if it's lower, it is possible that you have a sluggish thyroid. You may use the armpit temperature for ten minutes, but taking your oral temperature is just as effective. Be sure to add 1/2 degree to your oral temperature when comparing to the values above.

IS YOUR THYROID SLOW OR YOUR ADRENALS LOW? (OR BOTH?)

If you suffer from CRPS, it can be very difficult to tell whether you have tired adrenal glands or a slow thyroid gland. Telling the two apart can be a tricky business indeed. To further complicate matters, one will affect the other, and therefore, you may suffer from *both*. If you suspect either of these conditions, you really should get tested for both. However, I want to mention some of the most common symptoms more unique to each condition.

Putting Out the Fire

Please note that this list is merely meant to serve as a guide. It is not all-inclusive and should not serve as a definitive diagnostic tool.

We have discussed in depth what autonomic dysfunction does to your body. In the following chapters, we will examine *why* your autonomic nervous system is on the fritz and why the vagus nerve of CRPS patients malfunctions.

Tired Adrenals	Low Thyroid
Weight gain around the belly	Generalized weight gain
Temperature fluctuates	Temperature fairly steady
Hair fine and sparse	Hair coarse and sparse
Nails thin and brittle	Nails normal or thick
Sunken eyes	Skin around eyes puffy
Skin dry	Skin oily or moist
Full eyebrows	Sparse eyebrows outer 1/3–1/4
Retains fluids	Fluid retention normal
Ragland's blood pressure test positive	Ragland's test negative
Trembling	No trembling
"Smoothed out" fingerprints	Normal fingerprints

6

Slow Fire Burn: The Role of Inflammation in CRPS

The nervous system holds the key to the body's incredible potential to heal itself.

—Sir Jay Holder

A healthy body is the guest chamber of the soul; a sick body isits prison.

—Francis Bacon

When we think of inflammation, we think typically think of injuries, such as and inflamed ankle or an infection, sometimes as innocent as a pimple. We all know the signs of infection: heat, redness, and swelling. Chronic inflammation is quite a different animal, however. It is silent, for the most part, which is why it has been called "the hidden disease." It can wreak havoc on your internal organs and it can lead to serious health conditions, such as arthritis, cancer, and CRPS.

Chronic inflammation starts with the immune system. When you are injured or sick, your body sends an army of white blood cells to the site(s) of the infection. White blood cells are meant to kill off bad bacteria, malignant or cancerous cells, viruses, parasites or any other potential pathogens or foreign invaders that are capable of causing disease. These white blood cells respond to these invaders and kick start the healing process. In small doses, inflammation is crucial for your health: It helps to heal injury and infection. When you get an infection, like a cold, break a bone, or suffer any other sickness or injury, your immune system recognizes that your body is in danger and sends an army of inflammatory cells to fight foreign invaders. These cells rush to the site of injury or infection and release powerful chemicals to attack invading bugs.

As mentioned above, inflammation is the first response to an injury or infection, which causes a rush of blood plasma and immune cells to a targeted area. Injured tissues release a number of special signaling molecules which cause blood vessel dilation and increase blood vessel permeability, and causes cells that line the blood vessels to present adhesion molecules on their surface. These adhesion molecules are recognized by immune cells in the blood, which attach to the adhesion molecules, much like Velcro, and causes them to stick to the blood vessel walls. These signaling molecules now cause the immune cells to leave the blood vessel and move to the site of injury.

When harmful unwanted invaders are healed or killed, your inflammatory cells retreat, causing your immune system to calm down again and the inflammation to subside. However, the inflammatory cells don't always retreat. Sometimes they keep attacking, turning on your own body. This results in your immune system remaining in a state of constant stimulation, resulting in a chronic destructive inflammation. Your body was not designed to accommodate this type of faulty immune activity, and eventually, the army of white blood cells will start damaging the body from the inside.

When this happens, the immune system becomes misguided and is sent out on an unnecessary mission. The white blood cells are sent out to attack, but there is no enemy target. Those misguided white blood cells still mobilize just like they would if you were actually under the weather or suffering from an infection, but because there's no infection for them to attack, they end up just hanging around, often for years. You want your immune system to work like a focused sniper attack on viruses, bacteria, or cancer. But when you have chronic inflammation, your immune system works more like a sustained shotgun blast, damaging everything in its path. This may also cause damage to cells that your body needs on a daily basis to fight off diseases like cancer, leaving the body vulnerable.

ALL THE OTHER PLAYERS RESPONSIBLE FOR INFLAMMATION

Histamine

One of the best known inflammatory signaling molecules is histamine, which is capable of dilating blood vessels, increasing blood vessel permeability, allowing immune cells to leave the bloodstream and enter the damaged tissue.

Neutrophils

The very first immune cells that arrive at an injured site are neutrophils; a type of white blood cell that respond quickly to the site of injury or infection, and once there will recognize and destroy bacteria. Neutrophils are the most numerous types of white blood cells in the blood, and their job is to immediately respond to inflammation and kill bacteria by phagocytosis, a process by which these cells engulf, destroy and digest other cells, bacteria or cellular debris. Think of the old game Pac-Man, where invaders are simply "eaten up."

T-cells

T-cells are a type of white blood cells called lymphocytes. They are produced in the bone marrow, after which they spend some time maturing and developing in the thymus, a small organ with two lobes located in front of the heart, or inside the tonsils. Inside the thymus, 98 percent of T-cells will die by either positive or negative selection. After the lucky remaining 2 percent mature, they are located in the blood and in the lymph nodes.

T-cells are at the core of adaptive immunity, where your body is trained to recognize specific invaders and tailor its present and future plan of attack to it. T-cells are broadly divided into killer cells, circulating and scanning the body like soldiers on a mission, looking for cancerous or infected cells, simply by scanning their surfaces. These cells are then destroyed. The other type of T-cells are helper cells. These cells regulate different immune responses in the body. If there are methylation cycle problems or mutations in the body, as is the case in MTHFR abnormalities (see chapter 5), you may have trouble making the bases that are needed for new DNA synthesis. If you cannot make new DNA, then you cannot make new T-cells and as a result you may lack immune system regulatory cells.

Methylation also plays an important role in the ability of the immune system to recognize foreign bodies, pathogens or antigens that it needs to attack. Research has shown that methylation is decreased in humans with autoimmune conditions.

Macrophages

Macrophages are types of white blood cells formed in response to an infection or accumulating damaged or dying cells. They are large cells that are specialized to recognize, engulf and destroy the target cells. Think of macrophages as your body's garbage men. When a macrophage digests a microbe, it presents the microbe's antigen on its surface, serving as an alert system to other white blood cells. This causes the immune system to remember the invader, resulting in future responses to be more targeted and faster.

Cytokines

Cytokines are tiny diverse proteins produced by different types of immune system cells. Their function is to act like messengers between the cells of the immune system, regulating immune responses like the inflammatory response, immune response, and your body's response to cancer. Cytokines regulate the immune response in the body's fluids outside of the cells, as well as the immune response inside the body's cells. They act through receptors on cell membranes, as each cytokine has a matching cell surface receptor, much like a lock and a key. They also regulate the growth and excitability of certain immune cells.

Cytokines can even inhibit the action of other cytokines, or trigger the release of other cytokines. For this reason, cytokines are crucial in the over- or underresponse of the immune system, and play a crucial role in chronic inflammation. While generally good, cytokines may turn "rogue," becoming dysregulated and pathological. In this scenario, cytokines have been linked to many disease processes like rheumatoid arthritis, cancer, major depression, Alzheimer's, and CRPS.

When cytokines really become out of control, cytokines can trigger a dangerous reaction in the body known as a "cytokine storm," a reaction that occurs when the feedback loop in the immune response becomes unchecked by the body, and cytokines keep triggering the T-cells and macrophages to travel to the site of the infection, as well as causing more cytokines to be released. This reaction is often fatal.

Free Radicals

Free radicals are small destructive unstable molecules in your body that, like unwelcome squatters in your house, will destroy it from the inside out. While outside chemicals can cause free-radical damage, it can also come from *within* your body. When the mitochondria inside the cells create ATP (adenosine triphosphate, the fuel that drives the cells), they create free radicals as a by-product. Luckily, the body naturally has a mechanism to deal with these molecules. How? The body uses antioxidants to neutralize the free radicals. This is why we are urged to consume lots of fresh veggies and fruits, such as berries.

However, there is a catch. Due to the fact that most people don't eat healthy diets and therefore their bodies lack in nutrients, and the sheer overwhelming volume of chemicals we are exposed to from the environment, our bodies do not have enough antioxidants left over to neutralize both the free radicals created inside the cell naturally and the toxins we are bombarded with from the outside. The body uses glutathione to fight these toxins. However, it takes four ATPs to produce just one molecule of glutathione. In a sick body overwhelmed by toxins and already short on energy, this is a very expensive exchange that it cannot afford.

As a result, your cells are drowning in free-radical buildup like tiny cesspools. When cells are unable to keep up with housekeeping due to a lack of energy, the result is inflammation inside the cells, called intracellular inflammation.

Nitric Oxide (NO)

Nitric oxide (NO) is one of the most versatile players in the immune system, as a large number of immune cells respond to NO and also produce it to attack pathogens in various ways. Its role essentially is that of an intercellular messenger. It actually starts off the inflammation cycle. Macrophages, for instance, releases NO in order to inhibit pathogen replication. Think of NO almost as an Agent Orange of sorts, used by our own immune cells in the war against pathogens. It also regulates the growth, death, and functional activity of many inflammatory and immune cells.

NO has also proven itself to be a crucial factor in acute and chronic inflammation. NO gives an anti-inflammatory effect under normal physiological conditions. On the other hand, NO is considered as a pro-inflammatory mediator that induces inflammation due to overproduction in abnormal situations. In these situations, it has therefore been indicated in being a *pro-inflammatory* agent, meaning that it encourages inflammation.[23]

If your body is not equipped with enough antioxidants to get inside the cell and stop NO from increasing inflammation, it results in NO becoming like a freight train racing out of control, causing NO to combine with a free radical called superoxide. This results in one of the most toxic free radicals inside your body known to man to be created: peroxynitrite or ONOO. As if that isn't bad enough, ONOO has twenty-two different ways to create more NO, which in turn creates even more ONOO. This results in a vicious cycle like a wildfire raging out of control on a windy day. Our bodies need antioxidants to stop this vicious cycle.[24] In addition, when you suffer from the MTHFR gene mutation (chapter 5), your body will be depleted in glutathione. Superoxide rises because of glutathione depletion, which produces a rise in hydrogen peroxide (causing superoxide to rise).

MTHFR gene mutations can hurt you in other ways. Remember how it causes problems in the methylation cycle? As a result of the block in the methylation cycle, NO rises, causing lowered production of asymmetric dimethyl arginine, which is normally the main inhibitor of nitric oxide synthase. A partial methylation cycle block causes less production of this inhibitor, and that also allows nitric oxide to rise.

THE ROLE OF THE VAGUS NERVE

Let's talk about the anatomy of the vagus nerve in just broad terms. Deep inside the neck, a fibrous structure called the carotid sheath is located. The Carotid sheath is a fibrous structure that surrounds the vagus nerve, the internal jugular vein, and the carotid artery, essentially holding them together. The carotid sheath runs down the neck, and happens to be located just anterior to the lateral masses of the Atlas bilaterally. The lateral masses are two bulky masses of bone located on the sides of the ring shaped Atlas (uppermost vertebra), almost like ears. Therefore, any abnormal movement of the Atlas may affect the carotid sheath on one or both sides. Let's discuss the all-important Atlas vertebra in just a bit more detail.

THE ATLAS AND THE VAGUS NERVE

The Atlas is the very first bone in the spine. It is ring shaped and positioned right beneath the skull, where the brain stem turns into the spinal cord. This makes it a critical factor that may affect the central nervous system function. It is pretty much the portal to the entire spinal cord. It is also part of the most moveable joint in the body. Just think of all the ways you can move your head. The Atlas helps to make this possible.

Normally, this bone sits in a neutral position, held in place by various ligaments. It is not too forward, not too far back, nor rotated to one side or the other. However, when this bone moves from its normal position (called a subluxation), due to some kind of direct or indirect trauma or biomechanical stress, it may have devastating effects on the nervous system. Since the nervous system is the most basic system affecting every other system, organ and cell in the body, this will have a global impact on your health. The vagus nerve in particular, as mentioned above, is sensitive to misalignment of this bone. Misalignment of this very important bone in the spinal column is often part of the perfect storm resulting in the monster known as CRPS.

VAGAL TONE

Vagal tone is the internal biological process referring to the activity of the vagus nerve. Vagal tone may either be increased or decreased. It is possible for the vagus nerve to be compressed externally by malposition of the Atlas (as mentioned above), calcified or tight muscles or ligaments, and bone spurs (abnormal bony deposits in the spine, found when arthritis of the spine is present).

The vagus nerve may also be compressed internally. How does this happen? When the pressure in the internal jugular vein increases, it takes up more space in the carotid sheath. Since the carotid artery won't give (due to the high pressure of the blood flowing through it), the bulk of the pressure will affect the vagus nerve instead, since *something* has to give. I credit this discovery to Diana Driscoll, OD. Dr. Driscoll specializes in the treatment of POTS (Postural Orthostatic Tachycardia Syndrome) and EDS (Ehlers-Danlos Syndrome). You can read more about her work in The Driscoll Theory. Other things that may affect the pressure in the jugular vein are heart conditions (such as right-sided heart failure), lung conditions, or kidney failure.

It is also possible that infections may affect the vagus nerve. This infection may be present in the gut, or viral, such as herpes infection. The inflammation caused by an infection may adversely affect the vagus nerve, causing systemic inflammation in return.

VAGUS NERVE AND CRPS

As discussed in the previous chapter, if you suffer from CRPS, you suffer from an abnormally functioning vagus nerve. This may be a result of an injury to your upper cervical spine (neck) directly, such as a whiplash injury (discussed in chapter 7 in greater detail), or as a result of an abnormally functioning autonomic nervous system. Either way, malfunctioning of the nervous system is involved (by definition) when the vagus nerve is messed up. What does the vagus nerve have to do with inflammation? A lot, as you may guess.

Dr. Kevin Tracey, a neurosurgeon in New York, has done extensive research regarding this topic. Dr. Tracey set out to prove his hypothesis that the brain might be using the nervous system, and more specifically, the vagus nerve, to tell the spleen to switch off inflammation everywhere in the body. He derived at this idea after injecting an anti-inflammatory drug into a rat's brain in an effort to minimize the effects of a stroke. To his astonishment, he found that this action not only turned off inflammation in the brain, but turned off inflammation in the entire body.

If Dr. Tracey was right, inflammation in body tissues was being directly regulated by the brain. This was an extraordinary idea. Earlier, no one has ever really explored whether the cells of the immune system were being directly controlled by the vagus nerve. Now, it was emerging that it was entirely possible that the brain, via the vagus nerve, was the force that governed it all.

His first study involved cutting the vagus nerve in rats. When Tracey and his team injected the anti-inflammatory drug into the brain, the drug no longer had an effect on inflammation in the rest of the body. Viola! The second test was to somehow stimulate the nerve without any drug in the system. "Because the vagus nerve, like all nerves, communicates information through electrical signals, it meant that we should be able to replicate the experiment by putting a nerve stimulator on the vagus nerve in the brain stem to block inflammation in the spleen," he explained. "That's what we did and that was the breakthrough experiment."[25]

The vagus nerve works as a two-way highway, passing electrochemical signals between the organs and the brain. In chronic inflammatory disease, Tracey figured out, messages from the brain telling the spleen to switch off production of a particular inflammatory protein, tumor necrosis factor (TNF), weren't going through. Low vagal tone (or function) causes inflammation in the body. High vagal tone (or function) causes the reversal of inflammation.

Good communication between the immune system and the brain is therefore vital for controlling inflammation. The inflammatory reflex is a mechanism in which afferent (body to brain) vagus nerve signaling, activated by cytokines or pathogens, is functionally associated with efferent vagus nerve–mediated output to regulate pro-inflammatory cytokine production and inflammation. Vagus-nerve stimulation suppresses local and serum pro-inflammatory cytokine levels.[26]

Of course, the problem in the body of a CRPS patients is that (as discussed in chapter 5), the vagus nerve is anything *but* communicating with the body, and vice versa. It is much more like a traffic-clogged freeway, where few signals are making it through in either direction. Is it any wonder that CRPS patients are literally burning alive from the inside?

HOW CHRONIC INFLAMMATION CAUSES PAIN IN CRPS

Remember cytokines? It has been shown that certain cytokines are involved in not only the initiation but also the persistence of pathologic (abnormal) pain by directly activating nociceptive sensory neurons (nocireceptors are the nerves which sense and respond to parts of the body which are damaged). A good example of nociceptive pain is the pain experienced after burning.

Certain inflammatory cytokines are also involved in nerve injury (and inflammation-induced) central sensitization. We will discuss central sensitization in more detail in chapter 7. For now, just know that it fits the pain of CRPS to a T.

Certain inflammatory cytokines in dorsal root ganglion (or DRG, a collection of afferent sensory nerves that exists just outside of the spinal cord), injured nerves or skin are known to be associated with specific pain behaviors and with the abnormal spontaneous activity from injured nerve fibers or neurons. Following a peripheral nerve injury, immune cells that gather around the injured nerve(s) secrete cytokines. Localized inflammatory irritation of the dorsal root ganglion (DRG) not only increases pro-inflammatory cytokines but also decreases anti-inflammatory cytokines. There is abundant evidence that certain pro-inflammatory cytokines are involved in the process of pathological (abnormal) pain.[27]

SYMPATHETIC SPROUTING

Nerve sprouting is the process whereby nerve cells generate additional branches (outgrowths) to establish new synapses or to alter the strength of existing synapses, most often after nerve injury. In the nervous system, a synapse is a structure that permits a nerve cell (or neuron) to pass a chemical or electrical signal to another neuron. In animal models of pathological pain, abnormal sprouting of sympathetic fibers around large- and medium-size sensory neurons has been observed in dorsal root ganglia (DRG). Pro-inflammatory cytokines play a facilitating role in sympathetic sprouting induced by nerve injury, and its effect on pain behavior is indirectly mediated through sympathetic sprouting in the dorsal root ganglia (DRG).

Following peripheral nerve injury, sympathetic efferent fibers extensively sprout into both the DRG and spinal nerves. Sprouting fibers sometimes form distinctive basketlike webs (called sympathetic "baskets"), wrapping around DRG nerves. Pain induced by localized inflammation of the DRG or mechanical compression of the DRG in the absence of nerve injury can also be accompanied by sympathetic sprouting. Nerve sprouting usually causes proliferation of sensory nerve (in other words, instead of a nerve here and there, you now have a dense network of nerves).

SYMPATHETICALLY MAINTAINED PAIN (SMP)

The specific pain accompanied by hypersensitivity that CRPS patients suffer from is called sympathetically maintained pain (SMP). SMP is the result of efferent (away from the brain to the peripheral nerves) noradrenergic pain. Noradrenergic means that the nerves use norepinephrine, a neurotransmitter released by the sympathetic nervous system. Keep in mind that CRPS patients suffer from sympathetic dominance. Remember the schoolyard bully? SMP will sometimes respond well in the early stages to a nerve block, which is why CRPS patients are told that it is crucial to get treatment early on.

In addition, the evil monster, that is, SMP is created when there is abnormally enhanced communication between the sympathetic nervous system and the sensory nervous system. This enhanced communication may happen either in the central or peripheral nervous system. Pain induced by localized inflammation of the DRG or mechanical compression of the DRG in the absence of nerve injury can also be accompanied by sympathetic sprouting in the DRG.

PAINFUL TRIGGERS

Pain anywhere in the body, not directly related to the pain of CRPS, will usually amplify the pain caused by CRPS. I will give you a simple example: One of my favorite patients, Barbara, suffered from CRPS in her arm and hands. She also suffered from plantar fasciitis (inflammation in the bottom of her foot). When she walked long distances and her foot hurt, it would trigger her CRPS pain. After undergoing care in my office, her CRPS pain has been mostly under control (she now rates her pain at a 0–2/10, without medication). We also treated the plantar fasciitis extensively, as it seemed to be an active trigger of her CRPS pain. She occasionally still suffers from brief flares, after which time it will calm down again. Luckily, she also has times now when she has absolutely no pain. She can also walk long distances again.

Suffering from a cold, flu, or any other condition or disease will usually have the same effect. Stress in one part of the body affects the CRPS in another part. Again, if you view the body as a unit, this makes perfect sense.

THE DREADFUL SPREAD

It amazes me that so many doctors still do not acknowledge that CRPS may spread to other sites, when I have seen such clear widespread evidence of it in the CRPS community. This spread may happen even in the absence of a new injury, for apparently no logical reason at all. In my opinion, the general malfunction and continuous degeneration of the central nervous system, rather than a new injury, is most often to blame for this phenomenon. At least one study has pinpointed three possible patterns of spreading in the CRPS community:[28]

1) A "continuity type" of spread where the symptoms spread upward from the initial site, for example, from the hand to the shoulder
2) A "mirror-image type" where the spread was to the opposite limb
3) An "independent type" where symptoms spread to a separate, distant region of the body—this type of spread may be spontaneous or related to a second trauma

In my experience, understandably, few things strike fear in the CRPS patient's heart as the fear of the pain of CRPS spreading. Even if CRPS has seemingly gone into remission, patients usually still worry that it may recur. I often get panicked phone calls from CRPS patients after they have completed my treatment program, after they suffer a new injury. One of these patients even injured the same joint that originally gave rise to the CRPS (her elbow). Luckily, so far, not once has the CRPS spread in any of my patients post treatment. If the malfunction of the central nervous system is corrected, it seems to prevent the recurrence and spreading of CRPS.

OTHER POSSIBLE INFLAMMATION TRIGGERS OR CONTRIBUTORS TOXICITY

Why does a house get messy? There are two possible reasons, or usually a combination of both. The first reason is that you are too busy or overwhelmed to clean it. Things get put off (like vacuuming or folding laundry) and pile up. The other reason it may get messy is that you can't keep up with it, since it's being messed up faster than you can clean (if you have children, you probably know what I mean!) Think of your body as a house.

Every day, toxins enter your body and your "house" gets dirty. Toxicity causes widespread inflammation.

WHAT ARE TOXINS?

Toxins can enter our bodies from the external environment or be produced by us internally. Our body naturally produces internal toxins as a by-product of the metabolic functions it performs each day. Antioxidants are crucial in eliminating free radicals from your body. What exactly are free radicals? Free radicals are basically very reactive particles (small loose cannons, if you will) that move all around the cell damaging everything they come in contact with. Most are produced as a by-product of metabolism, but they can also arise from exposure to toxins, such as heavy metals.

In a nutshell, we are bombarded by toxins. When the body digests food, it produces toxins and waste. When it heals and repairs itself, it produces waste. Whenever we experience negative feelings like stress or anger, we also produce harmful toxins.

However, our bodies were designed to be able to naturally eliminate these toxins. We get into trouble when we are bombarded with the second kind of toxins, which are found in our food, water, and environment: human-made toxins. We eat them, drink them, breathe them, touch them, inject them, swallow them in our medications, and put them on our skins regularly and repeatedly. Our cells never get a break! We live in a toxic environment, and while you can control some aspects of your environment (such as the food you eat) it is impossible to avoid toxins altogether.

Consider this: according to the Environmental Protection Agency (EPA), four billion pounds of chemicals are released into the ground and hundreds of millions of pounds of chemicals discharged into surface waters such as lakes and rivers each year. In the United States, we allow more than ten thousand additives into our food supply. Each American eats an average of about 142 pounds of additives and toxins each year. Typically, eight pounds come from salt, 120 pounds come from sugar, and about fourteen pounds from coloring, preservatives, and flavorings. It is not a question of "if" we are toxic, but rather of how much it affects our health.

The body gets rid of toxins through breathing and sweating as well as through the colon, kidneys, and liver. When my patients mention a detox, they are most often thinking of a colon detox. However, the liver is incredibly overburdened and must not be ignored. Why may your liver be overworked? The liver performs over five hundred different tasks and is truly an amazing organ. However, your liver is essentially the filter of your bloodstream, and like any filter, it can become clogged with waste materials when it takes in more toxins than it can filter. When toxins overwhelm the liver, it can no longer perform as it should. Fat may accumulate in the liver or in other organs. Toxins build up and get into the bloodstream.

Among the signs of a toxic liver are weight gain (especially around the abdomen), headaches, bloating, indigestion, high blood pressure, elevated cholesterol, food allergies, memory loss, fatigue, acne, mood swings, depression, and even skin rashes. When the liver cannot do its work, the toxins that we are exposed to accumulate in the body and make us ill in an assortment of ways. They have damaging effects on many body functions, particularly the immune system. An overworked and undernourished liver is recognized as the root cause of many chronic diseases.

HEAVY METALS

Heavy metals include lead, mercury, cadmium, antimony, aluminum, arsenic, and many others. Many of the heavy metals, such as zinc, copper, chromium, iron, and manganese, are essential to body function in very small amounts. But if these metals accumulate in the body in concentrations sufficient to cause poisoning, serious damage may occur. Heavy metals enter our bodies in many ways. They may enter through cosmetics, amalgam dental fillings, water, improperly coated food containers and cookware, vaccinations, cigarettes, and many other things in our environment.

Symptoms of heavy-metal poisoning include anemia, fatigue, musculoskeletal complaints, mood disturbances, neurological problems, high blood pressure, gastrointestinal (GI) symptoms, kidney problems, liver dysfunction, endocrine problems, hormonal imbalances, and immune system dysfunction. Heavy-metal toxicity causes systemic problems that may fit the symptoms of many other syndromes. It presents in various body systems, depending on where the biochemical imbalance or disruption occurs, or the area(s) of highest toxicity of the metal(s)—for example, the brain, kidneys, or pituitary. Long-term exposure may contribute to the onset of slow progressive conditions such as Alzheimer's disease, Parkinson's disease, and cancer.

Laboratory tests routinely used for seriously exposed persons include blood tests, liver and renal function tests, urine tests, fecal tests, X-rays, and hair and fingernail analyses. Many of these tests are not routinely performed in your doctor's office. However, your physician can take blood samples and send them to the appropriate testing laboratory. While it is widely assumed that hair or fingernail analyses are best, I prefer blood or urine analysis. Hair and fingernail analyses can give an indication of exposure that has occurred over time or in the past but will not show recent exposures. Blood and urine will reflect exposures that are chronic or that have happened in the last few days.

Heavy-metal detoxification may be done in many ways. Many healthcare professionals use chelating agents. These include:

- **Dimercaptosuccinic acid (DMSA),** which, although being FDA approved, is mostly not recommended due to severe possible side effects, as well as unpredictable redistribution of mercury after being pulled from the kidneys, causing the mercury to be redeposited in the brain, kidneys, liver, or muscle tissue.
- **Ethylenediaminetetraacetic acid (EDTA)**, which is not a natural supplement. Like DMSA, EDTA is FDA approved. It has traditionally been used to treat lead poisoning. Unlike DMSA, EDTA is a weak chelator of mercury. Taking EDTA can be dangerous because it will chelate calcium and other essential minerals out of the body along with the toxic heavy metals.

- **Dimercapto-propane sulfonate (DMPS)**, an experimental drug used for chelation, is not approved by the FDA. Some doctors question the safety of this drug, pointing to the lack of research on its long-term effects on the human body.
- **Chlorella**, a variety of algae found in fresh water such as ponds or lakes. It is commonly used as a natural chelation supplement, meaning that it pulls out heavy metals such as mercury from the body. However, chlorella also pulls mercury from the water it is grown in, which naturally defeats the purpose of taking it in the first place. Analysis of at least one specimen of commercially available chlorella has shown high levels of mercury. You don't want to take a supplement riddled with mercury in order to remove mercury; that doesn't make sense.
- **Zeolite**, volcanic rock that attracts toxins and physically removes them from the body. Think of it as a taxi, loading up all the bad guys. Zeolite has a negative charge and a "honeycomb" structure with lots of holes. It is thought that this negative charge acts like a magnet and pulls the positively charged toxins, especially toxic metals, into the cells of the honeycomb, where the trapped toxins are then allegedly eliminated from the body through urine, sweat, and feces. However, no clinical trials have been done on zeolite and its effects on humans to date. Some animal studies have shown promise, and it is not a harmful substance, although some good minerals may be pulled from the body using zeolite. Mineral supplementation is recommended while using this product.
- **The ionic foot detox**, a footbath with an electric current. In a typical session the patient places his or her feet in warm salt water and an electrical array is turned on, creating electrolysis in the water. This electrolysis causes an electromagnetic field in the water that pulls toxins and heavy metals into the water through the sweat glands in the feet. During the session, the water changes its color and small floating particles appear. Although many people claim that the color change of the water is only due to oxidation and

that this method is a hoax; the truth is that 60 percent of the color change of the water is due to oxidation, and the other 40 percent is, in fact, due to the individual patient's toxicity, and will vary depending on the patient. I have personally seen notable and immediate reactions in my practice to this footbath, and I not only use it as part of my treatment plan but also use it personally twice a week.

- **Fasting and dietary detoxification**, generally consisting of cutting down on the number of calories you take in, eating very pure foods (consisting of lean organic grass-fed protein, raw nuts, and fruits and vegetables only, or juicing fruits and vegetables, or fasting and drinking lots of water). The general approach here is to provide the body with good nutrition while forcing it into ketosis, the process by which it is essentially burning its own fat for fuel. When the liver is overwhelmed, it does what any tired employee does—it puts its work off for later, to be detoxified when the liver isn't quite so busy. The body does this by depositing the harmful toxins in fat, sort of like a messy storage room. This protects the body and its valuable organs from these free-floating toxins. However, for many of us that day of detoxification never comes. When we fast, or reduce our calorie intake, the body will burn this dirty fat, and that day of reckoning and processing all those old toxins will finally arrive.

HEAVY METAL/CANDIDA LINK

By now, you have probably heard of the possible benefits of treating a candida or yeast overgrowth in the body. *Candida albicans* is a parasitic fungus that normally occurs in the gut, vagina, mouth, and other areas of the body.

Usually, candida is kept in check by your body's friendly or good bacteria. However, when the body is not well or when we take antibiotics that kill our friendly bacteria, this parasite will grow too rapidly and we may suffer from a host of different unpleasant symptoms, such as allergies, fatigue, sugar cravings, itching and burning, skin rashes, and many more. Candida can also damage the gut, leading to leaky gut syndrome. This will cause large particles to enter the bloodstream, in turn leading to autoimmune conditions and allergies (such as gluten intolerance) and affecting the brain and nervous system.

There are a variety of ways to kill a candida overgrowth in the body, one of which is to simply build up the body's good bacteria again. It is a very difficult infection to treat; it may take many months to get it under control in severe cases. However, a somewhat unknown but crucial piece of the candida puzzle that *must not* be ignored is possible heavy-metal toxicity. How are they linked?

Candida yeast serves the purpose of absorbing and sequestering heavy metals. Yeast overgrowth is one of the body's defenses to try and keep mercury and other heavy metals from damaging body tissues such as the brain. In other words, candida absorbs and binds mercury, thus protecting your body. As mentioned before, your body is infinitely smart. In its wisdom, it will choose a symbiotic relationship with the candida parasite over mercury toxicity. While candida is unhealthy, it is not as immediately damaging as mercury. Therefore, the body is choosing the lesser of two evils. When the uninformed patient or health-care professional then embarks on a war against candida, massive amounts of free mercury are released into the body, causing much more harm than good. If you suffer from a suspected candida overgrowth, it is therefore *crucial* that you get tested and treated for heavy-metal toxicity first. Be especially diligent if you have or have ever had amalgam fillings in your teeth.

THE DANGER IN YOUR MOUTH

Besides flossing, brushing our teeth, and getting professionally checked and cleaned a few times a year if we are diligent, most of us don't give our teeth a second thought.

I was first introduced to the importance of teeth while studying biological medicine. Biological medicine recognizes that the human being is a part of nature and reacts like everything else in nature. It seeks to awaken the healing powers that lie within us all through the use of natural methods and remedies. I was introduced to this work by one of my mentors, Thomas Rau, MD.

Dr. Rau is the medical director at the world's largest privately owned clinic, the Paracelsus Clinic (www.paracelsus.ch). The Paracelsus Clinic is located an hour away from Zurich, Switzerland, and employs about a hundred doctors, half of whom are dentists. People from all over the world come to this clinic to be treated for cancer, autoimmune conditions, and other conditions, often with astounding, unprecedented success.

Dr. Rau taught me that the teeth are linked to energy meridians, further linked to every organ in your body. It is crucial that the mouth be healthy. There is a reason why almost half the medical staff at this groundbreaking clinic are dentists. When patients enter care at the Paracelsus Clinic, their mouths are carefully examined.

Here are a few things that could be of concern in the mouth:

AMALGAM FILLINGS

If you have any silver-colored fillings in your mouth, this is usually a bad sign. A typical amalgam filling consists of approximately 50 percent mercury and 30 percent silver, as well as tin and copper. Mercury is a powerful poison. Published research demonstrates that mercury is more toxic than lead, cadmium, or arsenic. No amount of exposure to mercury vapor can be considered harmless, especially considering its cumulative effect.

In spite of numerous published scientific studies over the years demonstrating the ill effects of mercury fillings in the mouth, and considering that the FDA has never approved the amalgam mixture as a safe dental device, mercury/silver/amalgam fillings are still the primary material used by dentists in the United States (approximately one hundred million fillings are performed yearly).

The American Dental Association maintains that mercury is safe to use and harmless in the mouth, as the mixing of mercury is supposed to "bind" the mercury safely and render it harmless. However, electron microscopes have shown tiny droplets of mercury on the surface of amalgam fillings. Also, mercury vapors have been proven to escape these fillings and enter the bloodstream. Meanwhile, the World Health Organization has concluded that dental fillings contribute more mercury to the human body than all other sources combined.

Let's just ignore the controversy and look at a few facts about mercury: Mercury, before it is placed into the mouth, is a recognized hazardous toxin. The scrap amalgam that is removed from the mouth cannot simply be thrown away in the trash, or the dentist may be subject to a $10,000 fine by the Environmental Protection Agency (EPA). Instead, the scrap is considered a toxic waste and must be removed by a hazardous waste company in a specific way to keep the mercury from entering the water system.

It is crucial, if you have these fillings removed, that you have it done by an experienced dentist, as the removal is tricky and if done incorrectly may do more harm than good. Often the body is flooded with mercury during the removal process.

ROOT CANALS

A root canal is a common dental procedure that nearly every dentist will assure you is completely safe, despite the fact that scientists have been warning of its dangers for more than a hundred years. More than twenty-five million root canals are performed every year in this country.

Every day in the United States alone, approximately 41,000 of these dental procedures are performed on patients who believe they are safely and permanently fixing their problem. Sadly, the vast majority of dentists are oblivious to the serious potential health risks they are exposing their patients to, risks that persist for the rest of their patients' lives. The American Dental Association claims root canals have been proven safe, but they have no published data or actual research to substantiate their claim.

Teeth that have undergone root canals are dead teeth that can become dangerous incubators for highly toxic anaerobic bacteria. These bacteria could make their way into your bloodstream to cause a number of serious medical conditions, many of which might not appear until many years later. A tooth has one to four major canals. This is what is taught in dental school, and what is cleaned out in root canals. What is lesser known and often ignored by dentists and dental schools are the additional "accessory canals." A doctor named Weston Price did extensive research on these.

Dr. Price (1870–1948) was a dentist known primarily for his theories on the relationship between nutrition, dental health, and physical health. Dr. Price identified as many as seventy-five separate accessory canals in a single central incisor or front tooth. When we look at the structure of a tooth, we find three layers. First is the outer layer, known as enamel; then comes the second layer, known as dentin; and the inner part is the pulp chamber where the nerve resides. On the outside of the tooth is a ligament called the periodontal ligament, formed by fibers that come out of the tooth and intertwine with fibers coming out of the bone. Teeth are not actually attached directly to bone, but are attached by this ligament.

The second layer of the tooth, the dentin, is not really solid but composed of tiny tubules or canals. In a front tooth, if all these tubules were attached end to end, they would reach over three miles. Note that the tubules have adequate space to house many thousands of bacteria. Most of these toxic teeth feel and look fine for many years, which makes their role in systemic disease and inflammation even harder to trace back. In addition, these dead teeth may cause secondary infections in the bones of the jaw and face, not easily detected by the untrained eye on X-ray.

Many other problems can stem from teeth, such as other toxic materials or metals used in dental work, gum disease and infection, and the mixture of incompatible metals, such as gold fillings with certain metal fillings. If you suffer from CRPS or other chronic conditions, I urge you to have your teeth examined by a trained biological or holistic dentist.

The following organizations can help you to find a mercury-free, biological dentist:

- Consumers for Dental Choice
- International Academy of Biological Dentistry & Medicine (IABDM)

- Holistic Dental Association
- International Association of Mercury-Safe Dentists

CRPS PATIENTS BEWARE!

When it comes to patients suffering from CRPS, it is *very* important that great caution be taken when detoxifying. Even for a healthy individual, detoxification is very hard on all the organs and can cause symptoms such as headaches, muscle aches, fatigue, diarrhea, nausea, tremors, crying fits and anger, and many other side effects.

People who suffer from CRPS and probable MTHFR gene abnormalities are especially vulnerable to the side effects of detoxification, and their bodies are not always equipped to handle the stress of it.

We recommend that you only embark on a detoxification program with the help of a health professional experienced in detoxification.

HOW TO TEST FOR CELLULAR INFLAMMATION?

One of the best ways to tell if you have the condition is to get an hs-CRP test, a test that will detect C-reactive protein levels in the blood. C-reactive protein is produced by the liver and is elevated when inflammation is present anywhere in the body. It should not be present in high levels when there is no obvious sign of infection in the body. While this test is growing in popularity, is still not commonly administered or even understood by some doctors.

In our office, we use a simple, inexpensive urine test called the Meta-Oxy test to detect cellular inflammation. This test measures how much cell membrane damage is occurring in your body by measuring something called aldehydes, especially malondialdehyde, in the urine and is fifty times more accurate than a blood test. How does it work?

With trillions of cells in your body, this outer protective shell that holds the cell together and protects the cell is critical. It's literally where all communication takes place. The membrane is the real brain of the cell. Signals from our nervous system, endocrine system, and other cells in the body attach at this membrane and tell the cells what to do. This membrane not only plays a crucial role in telling the cell what to do, but also in allowing nutrients to enter the cell, and toxins to leave the cell. When the membrane becomes damaged, all the nutrition in the world, ingested by you through healthy foods, or supplements, cannot make it into the cells.

Every cell membrane in the body is made up of fat and cholesterol. The more cellular inflammation and damage that is occurring, the more fats are metabolized. The more malondialdehyde in the urine, the greater amount of cell membrane damage. This cell membrane damage is known as inflammation.

LET'S RECAP

This chapter contained a lot of chemistry, complicated processes and medical terms. Let's recap to make sure you understood (and will remember) the most important parts:

- Chronic inflammation causes chronic pain through various mechanisms, including something called sympathetic sprouting, as well as an abnormally sensitive communication between sensory nerves and the sympathetic nervous system.
- CRPS patients often suffer from MTHFR gene mutations. This will interfere with the nitric oxide cycle, which worsens chronic inflammation, as well as glutathione production.
- When you suffer from CRPS, your vagus nerve isn't functioning properly. This causes widespread inflammation of the body in various ways.
- CRPS patients tend to have a high level of toxicity and a difficult time detoxifying. This worsens chronic inflammation.

7

Pain, Your Dark Passenger

The worst kind of pain is when you are smiling just to keep the tears from falling.

—Hiro Mashima

I've had enough. I've seen enough, I want out, I want it to end, I don't care anymore!

—J. K. Rowling, Harry Potter and the Order of the Phoenix

There is no symptom more life-robbing to the CRPS sufferer than the constant, fiery, spirit-eroding pain. When you understand the mechanics behind the pain of CRPS, the pain makes perfect sense. Understanding the mechanics of your specific pain will bring you one step closer to hope.

TOXIC LESIONS OF THE DISC(S) IN THE NECK

Since the cervical spine, brain stem, and autonomic nervous system are connected, we should start with the nature of the original injury. When most people picture a disc injury, they think of a disc that was herniated, or "squished," and will show up as a big problem on an MRI. Sometimes, in their quest for answers, patients suffering from CRPS will undergo an MRI to rule out disc problems, because they often suffer from neck pain or frequent headaches (although this pain may be overshadowed by the pain from CRPS). It is very common for nothing noteworthy to show up on the X-ray or MRI, and the spine to then be dismissed as a problem. Patients are told that their spinal problems are "normal" for their age, that is, everyone seems to have them at that age. However, spinal degeneration is *never* normal just because it is common.

Sometimes, some of the most devastating disc injuries, in terms of the lingering and devastating effects they have on the body, may go undetected by normal imaging. A study performed on people who died from *nonspinal* injuries following car accidents and had "normal" MRIs and X-rays after these accidents proved this. All these people were found to have disc injuries that had been missed. These injuries included small tears, bulges, and fractures where the vertebra meets the disc.[29]

You may wonder why these small injuries matter. How can such a thing contribute to the development of CRPS? I credit the developer of a technology I use in my practice called frequency-specific microcurrent (FSM), Carolyn McMakin, MA, DC, for first introducing me to the following information:

Deep inside the discs of the spine (in the "nucleus" of the disc) is a neurotoxic substance called phospholipase A2, or PLA2. A small tear in the cartilage of the disc or in the surrounding parts of the disc will cause PLA2 to leak out into the spinal fluid, thereby exposing the spinal cord to it.

This nasty little substance has been shown to be so neurotoxic and inflammatory when present outside the disc that it will destroy the nerves it comes in contact with. We call this a "toxic lesion" of the spine. The part of the cord most likely to be damaged by this neurotoxic substance (the thalamic tract) just happens to be a part of the spinal cord that carries deep pain information. Usually, because of the location of the disc and this part of the spinal cord, the cord is unfortunately exposed to high levels of PLA2. This causes what is called "central pain," or "thalamic pain," which mimics nerve pain exactly. Central pain is different from the pain caused by the actual injury site where the CRPS originated. It is whole body pain that may accompany the pain of CRPS. You may say, it is additional pain.

Please note: If you have pain or aching in your hands and feet, regardless of where the pain of CRPS first originated in your case, you need to pay attention here. A very important benchmark of central pain is aching in the hands and feet.

SUBSTANCE P (THINK P FOR PAIN)

Nerve cells communicate with one another through messengers called "neurotransmitters." Substance P is one of these messengers. It is a protein found in the brain and spinal cord that is associated with some inflammatory processes in the joints. Its function is to cause pain. It essentially sends pain signals to the brain and spinal cord after it receives them from the sensory nerves. Interestingly enough, it has also been shown to be involved in increased stress and anxiety if elevated. The nerves that release Substance P have been shown to most likely be autonomic.[30] Severe or prolonged injury of these autonomic nerves will cause pain in different ways: parts of the spinal cord will become hyperexcitable, making them very sensitive to toxic stimuli, and these in turn will lower the pain threshold in the patient.[31]

CENTRAL SENSITIZATION

If you suffer from CRPS, you should care a lot about central sensitization. It is based on the principle that basically, pain itself may change the way the central nervous system works (meaning the brain and spinal cord), causing more pain, and causing the patient to become hypersensitive with less provocation. Sensitized patients are not only sensitive to things that would cause normal people pain, but also become sensitive to things that *shouldn't hurt*. Sound familiar? Any kind of noxious "bad" stimuli can trigger this reaction. Anything that hurts the skin, muscles, or organs. This pain can become constant and stick around even without provocation.

TWO PILLARS OF THE SAME BRIDGE: HOW TAILBONE OR LOW BACK INJURIES MAY AFFECT THE NECK

CRPS patients are all very fixated on the injury (or injuries) that triggered their CRPS. Whether it was something as innocent as a bunion surgery on the foot, or a devastating fracture, patients often live with what I refer to as the "if only" alternative story in their head. If only I didn't fall. If only I was more careful that day. If only I left that neuroma in my foot alone… the pain from it doesn't come *close* to the pain I live with now! Who can blame you? The truth is, though, that if not that injury, chances are that some other future injury would have eventually caused you to develop CRPS. Your body was most likely predisposed to it. The straw that broke the camel's back is not responsible for breaking the camel's back all by itself. It was merely the final action in a long chain of events leading up to it. Does this make sense?

One of the things that will put you most at risk for developing CRPS is cervical spine trauma, or low back or tailbone trauma. Think of the spine as a bridge with two stabilizing pillars on each end. If the low back or tailbone area becomes destabilized, the upper cervical spine will be affected too. In the spine, there is no such thing as an isolated injury. Every single part affects every single other part. For that purpose, we are about to cover this trauma in detail in the next chapter. Please do not mistake an injury to your spine with the same injury that triggered your CRPS (unless cervical spine or spinal cord trauma actually directly triggered it). In the vast majority, CRPS patients suffer from two separate physical injuries; spinal trauma (most often directly to the cervical spine, or indirectly to the low back or tailbone area(s)) that predisposes you to developing CRPS, and the injury (usually to a limb) that triggers it.

Many of my patients do not recall ever hurting their necks. However, these patients will often report injuries to their very low back or tailbone area(s). It may seem counterintuitive, as the atlas is at the very top of the spine, and the tailbone at the very bottom part of it. However, these patients have often suffered injuries (like a slip and fall on ice) or a tailbone fracture while giving birth. Think of the spine as a bridge with two stabilizing pillars at both ends. You cannot destabilize one pillar without it also affecting the other pillar. How exactly are these two areas directly connected?

We all have three membranes, called meninges, that surround the brain and spinal cord. These meninges are attached to the soft tissues and they form a three-layer cover that seals in the cerebrospinal fluid (CSF), much like Clingwrap (or Saran wrap, for my European readers). The meninges protect these delicate structures. The meninges are attached to the bony structures at the foramen magnum (the hole in the back of your skull where the spinal cord turns into the brain stem and attaches to the brain) and again at the sacrum (the flat triangular bone between your fifth lumbar vertebra and the tailbone). In between these two attachment points, the meninges are essentially free floating. If the coccyx is out of position, it will affect the way the sacrum moves. When the sacrum does not follow a normal moving pattern, it will create tension on these meninges, leading to dysfunction and misalignment of the upper cervical vertebrae in the spine.

While I don't expect that you become an expert in anatomy, it is also important to know that the upper cervical spine and the very lower sacral area both give rise to the parasympathetic (rest and digest) nerves. If you want to stimulate the parasympathetic nervous system (i.e., the vagus nerve), these are the areas that you will focus on. This is the case for CRPS patients, as it is vitally important to wake up the parasympathetic nerves and quiet the sympathetic nerves. For now, the most important thing I want you to take away from this information is that for CRPS patients, it is crucial that the bones in both your very upper cervical spine and your bones in the very lower spine (fifth lumbar, sacrum, and coccyx) are properly aligned.

While no exact percentages are known, it is my experience that the vast majority of patients who suffer from CRPS also suffered from upper cervical trauma or trauma to the very low back or tailbone area at some point. I would venture to put this number as high as 80 percent. For this reason, we are going to focus heavily on the involvement of these parts of the spine in CRPS.

It is important to note that the age of the injury is inconsequential. The mechanism of injury is often a car accident, but it can be attributed to many other mechanisms of injury, such as falls, birth trauma, or injury while under anesthesia (described in the "physical stress" section in the previous chapter). It is very important that you carefully examine your history from birth to adulthood when trying to understand what predisposed you to developing CRPS.

CERVICAL SPINE STENOSIS: DOES IT MAKE YOU VULNERABLE TO DAMAGE?

Since the genetic cause of CRPS is such a popular one, I want to introduce a possible link between the shape of the spinal cord, which may be genetic, and the predisposition for spinal injury following an accident.

Spinal stenosis is a narrowing of the open canal that surrounds the spinal cord, or the foramina (bony opening) where the nerves exit the spine. This can put pressure on your spinal cord and the nerves that travel through the spine. Spinal stenosis occurs most often in the neck and lower back. While some people have no signs or symptoms, spinal stenosis can cause pain, tingling, muscle weakness, numbness, and problems with bladder or bowel function.

It is postulated that two popular medications often prescribed for fibromyalgia and CRPS, Lyrica and Cymbalta, actually address the symptoms of spinal cord pain rather than the indirect symptoms of fibromyalgia or CRPS. The EU (European Union) approved Lyrica for central spinal cord pain. Of course, these medications simply address the *symptoms* of central spinal cord pain, and not the anatomical problem.

There are two types of cervical stenosis: congenital and degenerative.

CONGENITAL STENOSIS OF THE CERVICAL SPINAL CANAL

Some people are born with spinal stenosis. This is called *congenital stenosis*. They may not display any symptoms at a younger age, but having a narrow canal to begin with places them at risk for pain and injuries later in life. Even a seemingly minor neck injury can set them up to have pressure against the spinal cord. People born with a narrow spinal canal often develop problems later in life because the canal tends to become narrower due to aging, and the resulting changes in the spine. These changes often involve the formation of *bone spurs* (small bony growths caused by abnormal pressure in the spine) that put pressure on the spinal cord.

DEGENERATIVE STENOSIS OF THE CERVICAL SPINAL CANAL

Degeneration is the most common cause of spinal stenosis. Wear and tear on the spine from aging and from repeated stress and strain may cause many problems in the cervical spine. The intervertebral disc can begin to collapse, shrinking the space between vertebrae. Because of this collapse, bone spurs may form and protrude into the spinal canal, reducing the space available to the spinal cord.

Another common degenerative cause of stenosis is calcification of the posterior longitudinal ligament of the cervical spine. The posterior longitudinal ligament is situated within the vertebral canal. It extends along the posterior surfaces of the bodies of the vertebrae, or building blocks that form the spine, and goes down all the way to the sacrum, or the very lowest part of the spine.

All of these conditions may cause narrowing of the canal, leading to neurological symptoms and making you more vulnerable to spinal cord damage.

HOW DO I KNOW IF MY NECK IS THE PROBLEM?

Recognizing neck or upper back trauma in a CRPS patient can be tricky, since the majority of them either do not connect a past injury with their current diagnosis, or think that the injury was too insignificant to matter. Sometimes they may attribute it solely to the emotional stress that often accompanies a traumatic physical event, when both are actually to blame. I have seen this to be true especially in the case of domestic violence, where the emotional stress does play a role, but the physical injuries are dismissed as long healed.

There are a few clues that tend to point to spinal trauma as a culprit:

- A known past injury (or injuries) to the neck or upper back.
- Disc problems in the cervical spine, as seen on X-ray or MRI.
- Pain that does not respond well to medications or other treatments, such as massage therapy, physical therapy, surgery, trigger point injections, or exercise.
- Most will describe their extremities (hands and feet) as cold, aching, burning, or feeling as if they are "walking on glass."
- Severe headaches.
- The pain will start out more locally but will eventually affect the entire spine, especially low back, and eventually the whole body.
- Digestive problems.
- "Foggy" feelings and feelings of confusion. Vision, hearing, speech, smell, balance, or taste may be affected.
- Pain in shoulders and upper back.
- Pain in the jaw/TMJ.
- Central pain.

CENTRAL PAIN

What is central pain? WebMD defines it thus: "Central pain syndrome is characterized by a mixture of pain sensations, the most prominent being a constant burning. The steady burning sensation is sometimes increased by light touch. Pain also increases in the presence of temperature changes, most often cold temperatures. A loss of sensation can occur in affected areas, most prominently on distant parts of the body, such as the hands and feet. There may be brief, intolerable bursts of sharp pain on occasion."

This pain is sharp, stabbing, tingling, shooting, or aching, and affected by temperature changes.

WEATHER CHANGES

Why does your body respond violently to changes in the weather? When patients suffer from central pain syndrome (CPS), their nervous systems actually change on several levels. In CPS, nociceptors (tiny pain receptors) and peripheral nerves become hypersensitive. Pain amplification in the spinal cord tends to increase, and the spinal cord's ability to filter pain decreases. These changes become evident when the patient's sensory nervous system is exposed to any change, such as cold or heat or a drop in barometric pressure, which occurs when rain is coming in or the wind blows. This causes the sensory nervous system to respond to that change. Tissues will also swell as a result, making the patient's agony even worse.

There may be other reasons that bad weather makes you hurt. Donald A. Rhodes DPM, who designed one of the treatment systems I use in my clinic, called the Vecttor, has an interesting theory about why weather affects those who suffer from CRPS. According to him, ischemia (decreased circulation causing decreased available oxygen in the bone) leads to the accumulation of CO_2 in the affected tissues. This CO_2 combines with water to form carbonic acid, leading to a lowered pH. In bone, this decreased pH and oxygen are responsible for a breakdown of the bone matrix. This loss of bone leads to the formation of bone cysts. These cysts tend to show up in the area of increased oxygen usage, or beneath the cartilage, where muscles, tendons and ligaments attach. Eventually, the cartilage itself will begin to degenerate, leading to degenerative joint disease or arthritis. These bone cysts increase in size with low barometric pressure, leading to a profound increase in pain.

HOW CAN I BE TESTED?

Please remember that while several tests may show problems in the neck, most doctors are not aware of the link between spinal problems and CRPS. If you want to get clear answers about the health of your spine, you should probably not do so in the hope that it will affect your doctor's diagnosis or treatment of your CRPS. We do think it is very valuable information, especially on your road to understanding your condition and in searching for treatments that will work, and in finding eventual relief. Here are some of the tests that may uncover a link between your CRPS and cervical spine trauma.

CERVICAL X-RAYS

Although X-rays can be useful to show overall damage and misalignment of the bones and other structures of the neck, it is important to have a *trained eye* look at those X-rays. Typically, misalignments of the bones (such as the bone shifting abnormally to the front or the back, or twisting out of position) and loss of the C-shaped curve (or lordotic curve) of the neck are seen as "normal degeneration" of the spine by most allopathic doctors. Health-care professionals in the medical world are trained typically to not red-flag things that they often see and consider commonplace. Therefore, since degeneration is seen so often, it may be dismissed or only mentioned in passing.

A chiropractor is an example of a health-care professional who has been trained with the philosophy that the integrity and overall health of the spine are crucial to the overall health of the person, and who will look for clues that other radiologists or doctors may dismiss. It is not a question of competency, but rather training and overall philosophies about health in general.

The clues to be looked for may include decreased disc space, misalignment of the spine, and degeneration of the spine, which is abnormal bone growth that the body uses to stabilize weakened areas, like casting a broken bone. These bones may also fuse together, or you could have a decreased curve of the neck called a hypolordotic curve, which appears as a straight neck or one curved in the wrong direction (think of forcefully straightening a banana). Lastly, you may have a misalignment of the upper first two bones in the neck, called the atlas and axis, or a misalignment of any of the bones in the neck.

In chiropractic, this is referred to as "subluxation." The word "subluxation" is derived from the Latin word "lux," or light, where "sub lux" means less than light, or less than perfect. Chiropractors, often viewed by the public as "bone poppers," actually do so much more than that. They believe that the health of the spine is vital, given the importance of the central nervous system to the health of the overall individual.

The drawback of X-rays is that they are not good at showing the soft tissues—nerves, discs, and ligaments—and will not show the health or integrity of the disc clearly.

MRI

Magnetic resonance imaging allows health-care professionals to take a look inside your body at the soft tissue structures of the spine, such as the discs. According to Carolyn R. McMakin, MA, DC, a doctor who specializes in the treatment of the neurological symptoms of this type of fibromyalgia and CRPS, MRI studies of patients whose symptoms stem from spinal trauma will often show disc bulges (imagine a water balloon being squashed between two bricks). These disc bulges will most commonly appear between the fifth and sixth cervical bones or the sixth and seventh cervical bones, and less often between the fourth and fifth cervical bones.

Again, be aware that the average radiologist or doctor will see these changes as part and parcel of the "normal" aging process. Most MRIs are taken while the patient is lying down, which removes some of the normal weight that your discs carry when you are in an upright position. Although it is hard to find an imaging center that performs it, it is possible to do standing MRIs in the flexion (bending the neck forward) and extension (bending the neck back) positions, which will often show disc bulges that are "hiding" on conventional views.

FUNCTIONAL MRI
Functional magnetic resonance imaging or functional MRI (fMRI) is an MRI procedure that measures brain activity by detecting associated changes in blood flow. fMRI is used more in the research world than the clinical world. Although this technology is still in its infancy and not widely used yet, we did feel that it deserved a mention.

MYELOGRAM
A myelogram is an image that involves injecting contrast material by needle into the space around the spinal cord and nerve roots (the subarachnoid space) and then taking an image of it using a real-time form of X-ray called fluoroscopy. With the contrast material injected into this space, the radiologist is able to view and evaluate a very detailed picture of the status of the spinal cord, the nerve roots, and the meninges—the three membranes that cover the brain, spinal cord, and nerve roots.

The radiologist views the movement of contrast material in real time within the subarachnoid space as it flows and also takes X-rays of the contrast material around the spinal cord and nerve roots in order to show abnormalities in the spine. Although this type of imaging is very useful, injury to the soft tissues is always possible when a needle is used around the spine. For this reason, doctors prefer to order MRIs to view the spine.

PHYSICAL AND NEUROLOGICAL EXAMS
The CRPS patient will usually show abnormalities of the cranial nerves IX (the glossopharyngeal nerve) and X (the vagus nerve), diplopia (seeing one object as two objects, most often with one eye covered), hypersensitivity of the upper chest and lateral upper arms, poor balance or coordination, tingling in the arms and legs, and weakness of the arm and leg muscles.

The cranial nerves described above descend down from the cranium through the jugular foramen, which is right in front of the atlas. It is exactly in this narrow passage that something basically unknown to traditional medicine occurs: that is, the malposition of the atlas which can cause a pressure on the above-mentioned nerves, triggering pains that doctors fail to explain. As the vagus nerve lies almost in immediate contact with the transverse process of the atlas, rotary subluxation (malposition) of the atlas may cause pressure which can produce a wide range of symptoms.

Cervical trauma is sometimes not the only contributor to CRPS, but may be only one of the factors leading to "the perfect storm" we referred to earlier. In addition, patients who suffer from CRPS may often suffer from other conditions as well. In the next chapter, we will take a closer look at some of these.

8

As if CRPS Is Not Enough: Coexistent Conditions Adding to Your Misery

You can cut down all the weeds you want, but if you never pull the roots, they just keep coming back.

—UNKNOWN

There is a vast difference between treating effects and adjusting the cause.

—D. D. PALMER

Because CRPS is so painful, patients who suffer from it will mostly pay little attention to any other symptoms or health conditions they may be suffering from, in my experience. CRPS is like a blinding white light, obliterating anything else. I have often said that severe chronic pain will cause almost a numbing effect in the person who suffers from it. I have dubbed this a "pain callus." Patients who suffer from CRPS experience pain differently from other people. I always tell my patients that I'm a great example. The closest to your misery that I have ever felt was natural childbirth, which had an end. If I get the smallest headache (which happens maybe once a year), I will easily rate it at a seven to eight out of ten. I'm a wuss when it comes to pain! The average CRPS patient will barely blink at even a migraine. I believe that this phenomenon is not yet clearly understood, but that the body adapts to pain to some extent in order to survive, or it would drive you to insanity.

Once the CRPS patient recovers, their pain response will also return to normal, and do so rapidly. While this is often experienced as a loss by CRPS patients in my experience, it is vastly important to once again experience pain normally. Why? Your body uses pain and symptoms as an alarm system. If your brain cannot "hear" the alarm, it cannot be alerted to the problem. While you are suffering from CRPS, and you have this "super power" that allows your brain to ignore pain and other symptoms that simply cannot compete with the raging pain of CRPS, you may not pay attention to what is commonly referred to as "co-concurrent" conditions, which are conditions you suffer from in *addition* to CRPS. These conditions may also harm your health, and definitely deserve your attention.

When you go to your doctor, these conditions may be addressed, but typically they will be treated as separate and often unrelated to CRPS. However, remember—your body is a whole, not an engine made of separate parts. Every part affects every other part. Because of the complexity of the dysfunctional nervous system responsible for CRPS, the patient will often suffer from other conditions and symptoms also related to the same dysfunctional nervous system. Because your health is precious, it is important to understand what these conditions may be, so that the underlying cause may be addressed. Please understand that this topic alone could fill a book. Therefore, I cannot possibly touch on every single condition that may be related. I will attempt to cover all the big ones, though.

ALLERGIES

Patients who suffer from autonomic dysfunction (all CRPS patients) will usually also suffer from autoimmune dysfunction. The immune system is directly governed by the autonomic nervous system, and cannot function properly without it. Autoimmune dysfunction will usually eventually lead to autoimmune conditions, one of which is allergies. This causes a vicious cycle, as the more things you become allergic to, the more these foods or substances will cause inflammation when you consume them or are exposed to them. The vast majority of my CRPS patients will actually test allergic to their own body fluids, such as blood, saliva, and urine. Patients may even become allergic to their own sperm or vaginal fluid, or that of their partner. This will often result in unexplained infertility. It is foolish to treat the allergies, without first treating the autoimmune component, and in turn, the autonomic dysfunction underneath it all.

CHRONIC FATIGUE SYNDROME

As you may guess, the name of this syndrome says it all. When you suffer from this you are chronically, debilitatingly tired, and no readily apparent underlying medical cause can be found. Sleep becomes an obsession, but in a cruel twist, does not relieve your fatigue. This syndrome is usually only considered to be an "official" diagnosis once you have been fatigued for six consecutive months or more. It is often missed in CRPS patients because severe pain usually affects the quality and quantity of your sleep anyway.

CFS patients may also suffer from headaches, a weakened immune system, depression, increased sensitivity to light, sounds, and smells, digestive issues, and possible cardiac problems (all of which symptoms are also often found in those who suffer from CRPS). Physical or mental stress may make this syndrome worse. Patients who suffer from this should have both their adrenal and thyroid function thoroughly tested.

It is my belief that an unbalanced autonomic nervous system is responsible for the majority of cases of chronic fatigue syndrome, as the parasympathetic (resting and digesting) system is turned off and the sympathetic (fight-or-flight) systems are "on" all the time. Adrenal support and supplementation are crucial for these patients, as is balancing the autonomic nervous system so that the parasympathetic nervous system is turned back on.

DIGESTIVE DISORDERS

Because of the vagus nerve malfunction, CRPS patients almost universally will exhibit some form of GI symptoms or conditions. These symptoms may be as mild as constipation or as severe as gastroparesis, a complete shutdown of the GI system. Other diagnoses may include IBS (irritable bowel syndrome), diverticulitis, celiac disease, Crohn's disease and gluten intolerance, to name but a few.

In my experience, few doctors will treat these problems as a central nervous system dysfunction. It is far more likely that these patients will be prescribed medicine to counteract their symptoms. If they experience heartburn, they will be given antacids. If they are constipated, they will be prescribed medication for that. Of course, this complicates the toxic load your GI system is already dealing with, not to mention your liver and kidneys.

The following may cause digestive symptoms (especially in patients suffering from CRPS):

- Autonomic (parasympathetic) nervous system dysfunction, turning "off" digestion and the immune system in the gut, specifically malfunction of the vagus nerve
- Overuse of antibiotics causing an imbalance in good versus bad bacteria
- Candida overgrowth resulting from a weakened immune system, heavy-metal toxicity, or not enough good bacteria in the gut
- A poor diet low in fiber, acidic in nature, and high in sugar and saturated fats
- Medications adversely affecting the gut
- Weakened digestive enzymes, resulting in food not being completely digested
- Food sensitivities or allergies

The health of your digestive system is directly linked to the health of your immune system. Almost 70 percent of the immune system resides in your intestinal tract.[29] This branch of the immune system, made up of billions of friendly bacteria and yeast, is responsible for many functions including proper nutrient absorption, production of vital nutrients (produced by the bacteria in your gut), detoxification and alkalization of the body, and last but not least, one of the main weapons your body uses in fighting against bad bacteria.

While we do not have the luxury of space to discuss every digestive problem or diagnosis in detail, we feel strongly that the digestive system of every patient suffering from fibromyalgia must be treated as if it is not well.

THE BASIC STEPS NECESSARY TO HEAL THE DIGESTIVE SYSTEM

1) Detoxify
2) Avoid foods that you are allergic to (or get treated for your specific allergies)
3) Change your diet (please refer to chapter 11)
4) Rebuild the gut with good food and good bacteria
5) Nourish the body with healthy and proper vitamins, minerals, and supplements (please refer to chapter 12)

Every patient who suffers from CRPS should rebuild and restore their digestive system.

FIBROMYALGIA

(For more about this topic, please read my book; *Taming the Beast: A Guide to Conquering Fibromyalgia*). Fibromyalgia is a condition that causes the patient to experience chronic pain affecting the entire body that may "jump" from area to area, along with severe, chronic fatigue. Patients who suffer from fibromyalgia often will report that they suffered from some type of old cervical or tailbone injury, such as whiplash or falls. Like CRPS, fibromyalgia is neurologic pain. There is actually much overlap between these two conditions, although the pain experienced by CRPS patients is much more intense in nature than that associated with fibromyalgia. CRPS usually confines to one area, unless it spreads. It is possible, and in fact not uncommon, to suffer from both conditions at the same time.

RHEUMATOID ARTHRITIS (RA)

The vagus nerve is responsible for inhibition of pro-inflammatory cytokines (remember those evil little suckers from chapter 6?). It has been found that implanting a device that stimulates the vagus nerve often reverse the symptoms of RA within a very short period of time. Again, it seems that the vagus nerve falling down on the job is implicated. For this reason, many patients who suffer from RA may develop CRPS or vice versa. RA causes pain in the feet and hands and other joints in the body, and may deform those joints over time. RA is usually symmetric, unlike osteoarthritis, which may only affect a joint on one side, and results from wear and tear or old injuries. RA is an inflammatory autoimmune disease where your own body mistakenly attacks itself. It usually begins after age forty, but may affect even younger people. My CRPS patients who respond well to treatment often notice a dramatic change to their RA as well.

POST-TRAUMATIC STRESS DISORDER (PTSD)

Once called shell shock, PTSD is a serious condition that can develop after a person has experienced or witnessed a traumatic or terrifying event in which serious physical harm occurred or was threatened. PTSD is a lasting result of a traumatic experience that caused intense fear, helplessness, or horror, such as a sexual or physical assault, the unexpected death of a loved one, or an accident, war, or natural disaster.

Most people who experience a traumatic event will have reactions that may include shock, anger, nervousness, fear, and even guilt. These reactions are common, and for most people they go away over time. However, for a person with PTSD, these feelings continue and may even increase, becoming so strong that they keep the person from living a normal, happy life. People with PTSD have symptoms for longer than one month and cannot function as well as they did before the event occurred.

Patients who suffered sexual or physical abuse suffer from a high burden of stress upon their nervous systems and bodies, affecting the autonomic nervous system (as one perpetually lives in a state of fight or flight) and are much more likely to develop chronic conditions such as CRPS. Inversely, because of the trauma associated with suffering from high levels of daily pain, CRPS patients may sometimes develop PTSD *because* they suffer from CRPS.

MULTIPLE SCLEROSIS (MS)

Multiple sclerosis (MS) is a chronic, often disabling disease that was previously thought to be caused when the body's immune system attacks its own central nervous system (CNS), resulting in the myelin sheaths (think of them as insulation around electrical wires) around nerve cells in parts of the brain and spinal cord being damaged, in turn leading to loss of myelin and scarring. These changes affect the ability of nerve cells to communicate, resulting in a wide range of signs and symptoms. These symptoms may be mild, such as numbness in the limbs, or severe, such as loss of vision or paralysis.

The progress, severity, and specific symptoms of MS are somewhat unpredictable and may vary from one person to another. Typical symptoms may include fatigue, loss of vision or hearing, double vision or visual blurriness in the central visual field that affects only one eye, weakness of the arms or legs, neuropathy (tingling, pain or numbness) in the limbs, speech impairment, difficulty balancing, and bowel or bladder incontinence.

A diagnosis is often made after a careful history and neurological exam (the skills of the neurologist are crucial here), a spinal tap, blood tests (to rule out conditions with similar symptoms), MRI (to show lesions), and a neurological test called an evoked potential test (to show nerve damage).

The model for immune system dysfunction leaves one obvious question unanswered: *why* does the immune system turn on itself in the first place? After all, this seems to be a common occurrence in multiple conditions including MS, fibromyalgia, lupus, and rheumatoid arthritis. All share an immune system gone haywire and now on the prowl, damaging its own body. Since the immune system is governed by the central nervous system, it would make sense that there might be a link between this system and the immune system's nutty behavior.

A groundbreaking study performed in 2011 using upright MRIs found: *"Multiple sclerosis may be bio-mechanical in origin wherein traumatic injuries to the cervical spine result in cervical pathologies that impede the normal circulation of CSF to and from the brain."*[30] In layman's terms, this means that multiple sclerosis may also be caused by injuries to the cervical spine, such as car accidents. While more studies are needed, we find this research eye-opening and very promising indeed. In our work, we have noticed great changes in the neurological symptoms of MS when the upper cervical spine was treated and corrected.

LYME DISEASE

If you have Lyme disease, or know someone with Lyme disease, hang on to your chair, as we are about to give you a whole new look at this disease.

The most accepted and universal belief is that Lyme disease (Lyme Borreliosis) is an infectious tick-borne disease caused by at least three species of bacteria belonging to the genus *Borrelia*. Early symptoms may include fever, fatigue, headaches, or depression. A characteristic circular skin rash called erythema migrans (EM) appears around the bite. Left untreated, later symptoms may involve the heart, joints, and central nervous system. In most cases, the symptoms are eliminated by antibiotics, if treated early. However, delayed or inadequate treatment can lead to more serious symptoms, which may be disabling and difficult to treat.

Lyme disease is divided into three stages. First is early localized infection, where the infection has not yet spread throughout the entire body. During this stage, roughly 80 percent of patients will develop the characteristic "bulls-eye" rash at the site of the bite. The second stage is the early disseminated infection, when the infection spreads through the bloodstream within days to weeks after the onset of the initial local infection. This happens in only one in three hundred to four hundred cases, where again only 10 to 15 percent of patients may subsequently develop neurological symptoms such as meningitis (an infection of the membranes around the brain and spinal cord), shooting pains, and palsy of the face (where the muscles in the face become paralyzed).

Late disseminated infection (stage III) may occur after several months, when a small percentage of patients (about 5 percent) go on to develop severe and chronic symptoms that affect many parts of the body. This may include the brain, nerves, eyes, joints, and heart. Other serious symptoms may include "frank" psychosis, arthritis, vertigo, and bladder problems.

The current theory about Lyme Borreliosis was formulated in 1977. At that time, Allen C. Steere, MD, and his colleagues, who were studying rheumatology at Yale University (he is now a professor at Harvard), discovered a "new disease" called Lyme Borreliosis after substantial prospective trials. In 1983, the first international conference on Lyme disease took place at Yale University. However, in 2012, Dr. Steere stated that long-term symptoms seen in Lyme disease were, in his opinion, caused more by an immune system failure rather than an infection, and would not benefit from antibiotics.

The problem with the current Lyme disease theory is that not all people bitten by an infected tick become sick with Lyme disease. Therefore, it stands to reason that the immunity of the host must have something to do with it, and all the problems can't be caused by bacteria alone (we come full circle, once again back to the immune system). It follows then that part of a well-rounded treatment program should be to strengthen the body and immune system from the inside.

TREATMENT STEPS FOR LYME DISEASE

It is our opinion that unless the infection is less than two weeks old, it should not be treated with antibiotics. Please find a health-care practitioner knowledgeable in Lyme disease who can guide you through the following treatment steps:

1) Get tested for heavy-metal toxicity.
2) Detoxify your body of all toxins.

3) Improve the overall health of your body with diet, supplementation, and specific treatments aimed toward improving the immune system.

Lab testing will rule in or rule out Lyme disease in most cases.

Tests include the Borrelia-DNA via PCR (polymerase chain reaction), which may be used to diagnose an acute infection in the first few weeks, but has proven to be rather inaccurate after that. If a suspected infection is older, an enzyme-linked immunosorbent assay (ELISA) test to look for IgG and IgM antibodies (which may give false negatives early on) or a Western blot test may be used.

INTERSTITIAL CYSTITIS (CS)

Interstitial cystitis (IC) or painful bladder syndrome (PBS) is a chronic inflammation of the bladder wall that causes nagging pain and severe discomfort. Symptoms often include a sense of urgency and increased frequency of urination. While a healthy adult urinates on average about six times a day, a person with IC may urinate up to seventy times in twenty-four hours, including several times at night, interrupting their sleep.

Inflammation associated with IC causes the lining to scar and the bladder to become stiff and less elastic, which may affect the way the bladder can expand. In about 90 percent of IC cases, there are pinpoint spots of bleeding visible in the lining. In up to 10 percent of cases, ulcers known as Hunner's patches may form on the bladder wall. As if this condition isn't uncomfortable enough, it may also worsen during menstruation and can cause intercourse to be painful for both sexes.

A large survey of 6783 patients with IC/PBS found that 40 percent of patients with IC also suffered from allergies, while 30 percent suffered from irritable bowel syndrome.

Cranberry extract (not juice) has proven to be somewhat successful, as well as a supplement called D-mannose. D-mannose is a type of sugar that has been shown to relieve IC/PBS. It is theorized that D-mannose might treat the deficiency caused by a genetic defect that causes abnormal breakdown and production of mannose or that D-mannose might prevent certain kinds of bacteria from sticking to the walls of the urinary tract and causing infection. (This supplement can be ordered at mercola.com.)

Interestingly enough, as if following a trail of breadcrumbs, the newest research again points to the autonomic nervous system as a direct cause of IC/PBS, where it is shown that people with IC/PBS also exhibit an overactive sympathetic nervous system.[31]

TRIGEMINAL NEURALGIA

Trigeminal neuralgia (aka tic douloureux) is a nerve disorder that causes sharp, sudden, searing, electric-shock-like facial pains and affects about one out of every fifteen thousand people, although it is much more common among those who also suffer from CRPS. The pain comes from a cranial nerve called the trigeminal nerve and usually affects one side of the lower face and jaw, although symptoms may appear near the eyes, ears, nose, jaw, or lips. Many experts say trigeminal neuralgia is the most unbearably painful human condition, and for this reason, it is tragically also known as "the suicide disease."

Trigeminal neuralgia has been linked with autonomic nervous system dysfunction.[32] In addition, at least one study has linked it to upper cervical trauma such as whiplash injuries.[33] Medically, this condition is treated with medications or surgery. We believe that this condition must be approached in such a way that the autonomic nervous system dysfunction is balanced and corrected. In addition, we correct any upper cervical misalignment and rehabilitate the trigeminal nerve in our treatment approach.

RESTLESS LEG SYNDROME

Restless leg syndrome (RLS) is a neurological disorder characterized by unpleasant sensations in the legs (and sometimes other parts of the body such as arms, trunk, or head), and an uncontrollable or overwhelming urge to move them. People with RLS may constantly move their legs (or other affected parts) to minimize or prevent these sensations.

Symptoms may include throbbing or a pulling and crawling sensation occurring primarily at night. Resting or lying down actually worsens these sensations, making it particularly disruptive to sleep and rest. The sensations range in severity from uncomfortable to irritating to painful. RLS is very common and may affect up to 10 percent of the population, especially the CRPS population. Medically, this condition is usually addressed through medications. At least one study has found a definitive link between sympathetic nervous system dysfunction and RLS.[34]

EHLERS-DANLOS SYNDROME

Ehlers-Danlos syndrome is a group of disorders that affect the connective tissues that support the skin, bones, blood vessels, and many other organs and tissues. Abnormalities in connective tissues cause the signs and symptoms of Ehlers-Danlos syndrome, which vary from mildly loose joints or hypermobile joints to life-threatening complications.

People who have Ehlers-Danlos syndrome usually have overly flexible joints and stretchy, fragile skin. A more severe form of the disorder, called vascular Ehlers-Danlos syndrome, can cause the walls of your blood vessels, intestines or uterus to rupture. Because this syndrome may affect the internal jugular vein, causing it to take up more space in the carotid sheath, it may put pressure on the vagus nerve, resulting in autonomic dysfunction leading to CRPS.

POSTURAL ORTHOSTATIC TACHYCARDIA SYNDROME (POTS)

When a patient's heart rate speeds up 30 beats per minute or more without much change in blood pressure on standing, the patient may have POTS. POTS is most frequently seen in young women, often less than 35 years of age. The increase in heart rate is usually a sign that the cardiovascular system is working extra hard to maintain blood pressure as well as blood flow to the brain.

Typical signs and symptoms of POTS include (but may not be limited to), profuse and sudden sweating, headaches of a throbbing quality, fainting, nausea, shortness of breath, exhaustion, chest pain, weakness, and visual changes. Once again, POTS is caused by an abnormally functioning autonomic nervous system, specifically indicating the vagus nerve. Often, the patient will report a viral infection shortly before the development of their symptoms. Remember, viral infections may directly inflame the vagus nerve.

VULVODYNIA

Vulvodynia is unexplained pain in the vulvar area (external female private part) or vagina, which can last for years. The pain that is its hallmark has been described as sharp, burning, rawness or stinging, much like dozens of tiny paper cuts in your private parts (yikes!). It affects approximately 16 percent of all females at some point and is therefore considered to be quite common. It is often made much worse by touch or indirect contact, making intercourse and wearing tampons darn near impossible. Traditional treatments are varied and typically not spectacularly successful. Once again, inflammation of the nervous system seems to be linked to this condition,[35] and stimulation of the vagus nerve seems to have a very positive effect on this condition.[36]

WEIRD CHEST PAIN

CRPS patients often suffer from atypical chest pain, which is more frequent in females than males. The cause of this is irritation and sensitization of the intercostobrachial (ICB) nerve. This nerve originates from the second intercostal nerve root (T2, or second thoracic vertebra) bilaterally from the spine and also has input from the T3 and T4 nerve roots. It supplies the axilla (underarm area), medial and anterior arm, and contributes to the innervation of the chest wall in the upper front area. It also contributes to the nerve supply of the back of the forearm and occasionally also the pectoralis major and minor muscles.

CHANGES TO YOUR BRAIN

Studies have shown that patients who suffer from CRPS show clear changes to the brain.[37] These changes included atrophy (or shrinking) of the gray matter (outside of the brain) and connectivity in the white matter (inside of the brain). The areas affected results in changes to the intensity and duration of pain; two things that CRPS patients can scantly afford. The changes in the brains and central nervous systems of CRPS patients may affect them in other ways, too. Severe neuropathic chronic pain has been shown to be associated with poor performance on neuropsychological tests that assess working memory, language, and executive function.[38–40]

While the above list is not all-inclusive, it covers many of the other symptoms that CRPS may suffer from. Keep in mind that an abnormal autonomic nervous system (ANS) may affect all kinds of other systems in the body. Whatever you suffer from, always try to trace it back to the central nervous system, thinking about your symptoms in a logical way, instead of just allowing your doctor to treat the symptom with a drug.

Speaking of drugs, let's delve into the traditional approach of the diagnosis and treatment of CRPS.

9

The Old Way: Current Diagnosis and Treatment Methods of CRPS

There is a vast difference between treating effects and adjusting the cause.

—D. D. Palmer

The best doctor gives the least medicines.

—Benjamin Franklin

THE MOST CONFUSING PART: OBTAINING A DIAGNOSIS

It is very difficult to find a doctor who is knowledgeable in recognizing and correctly diagnosing CRPS. Except for the lucky few, most CRPS patients may go many months or even years before they are correctly diagnosed with CRPS. If caught early, before brain, nerve and tissue changes set in, it is much easier to treat CRPS. For this reason, it is a true tragedy that some patients have to fight so hard to obtain a proper diagnosis. Although there is no one single definitive test for CRPS, there are a few things doctors look for when diagnosing this condition, and tests that help them to do so. If a patient is lucky, they will cross paths with a doctor well trained in the diagnosis and treatment of CRPS (most often a neurologist or anesthesiologist).

If a physician or physical therapist is not familiar with spotting or treating CRPS patients then this may sometimes result in serious problems and setbacks. CRPS is one of those diseases where doing the wrong thing is often worse than doing nothing. Like I mentioned above, the first year after the symptoms of CRPS first present themselves is like a golden window, as it is much easier to beat CRPS into remission during this period. After time goes by, certain physiological and anatomical changes make it a bit more challenging to beat the monster.

Diagnosis of CRPS is based on a physical exam and your medical history. Again, there's no single test that can definitively diagnose CRPS, but the following procedures may provide important clues:

THE THREE-PHASE BONE SCAN

The three-phase bone scan has been used since the mid-1970s to diagnose CRPS. An intravenous (IV) injection of a particular radiolabelled substance that has a special tendency to concentrate in the bones is administered and a technician takes images of the body part in question, looking for the initial phase of "blood flow." Immediately, he will look again for the second phase of "blood pool." Finally, approximately two hours later, images will show the concentration of the radiolabelled material in the actual bones; this is the "delayed phase."

It has been observed that there is a characteristic pattern of activity in the involved CRPS limb, which in the early 1980s was described as "pathognomonic"—a sign or symptom upon which a diagnosis can be made in this case of CRPS. There are some drawbacks to this test. There is no available data on how many of these patients who had a limb trauma, but no CRPS symptoms, had an abnormal bone scan as well. In addition, only 16 percent of the patients diagnosed with CRPS eight weeks after trauma had the characteristic bone scan pattern. To add to the confusion, a sympathectomy itself produces a pathognomonic CRPS bone scan. A sympathectomy is the removal of a single sympathetic nerve, or a group of sympathetic nerves in order to relieve pain. Many patients who suffer from CRPS have had this procedure done.

X-RAYS
X-rays are often used to diagnose complex regional pain syndrome (CRPS). X-rays may be used to identify signs of CRPS in the bone, such as loss of bone minerals, common in CRPS. X-rays may also be used to rule out other conditions which may potentially contribute to the patient's symptoms. As with several other diagnostic tools, X-rays typically cannot act as a stand-alone tool in the diagnosis for CRPS. Therefore, X-rays are often used in conjunction with other forms of diagnostic testing.

CRPS AND BONE LOSS
It is common for patients with CRPS to experience a decrease in bone mineral density. This bone loss typically occurs in the later stages of CRPS, three to twelve months after the onset of the condition. X-rays will typically appear normal during the first three months of CRPS. When CRPS affects the patient's bone, osteopenia occurs. Osteopenia is a condition that causes lower-than-normal bone density. In many cases, osteopenia is considered a precursor to osteoporosis.

THERMOGRAM
A thermogram is a noninvasive means of measuring heat emission from the body surface using a special infrared video camera. It is one of the most widely used tests in suspected cases of CRPS. As noted, detecting an abnormal change in skin temperature in CRPS depends on many factors. A normal thermogram does not necessarily mean the patient does not have CRPS. An abnormal thermogram may, however, be helpful when there are minimal objective findings for a diagnosis of CRPS documented in the medical record. Furthermore, certain patterns of abnormal heat emission from the body (e.g., circumferential versus dermatomal changes) are more indicative of the existence of CRPS than others. The thermogram

should be performed at a reputable medical facility. The quality of the test may vary among providers.

About 80 percent of CRPS patients have differences in temperature in opposite sides that may be either colder or warmer. These temperature changes may be associated with changes in skin color. Furthermore, the temperature differences are not static. The skin temperature can undergo dynamic changes in a relatively short period of time (within minutes) depending critically on room temperature, local temperature of the skin, and emotional stress. In some cases, the differences in temperatures may fluctuate spontaneously even without any apparent provocation.

NEUROLOGIC TESTS

The typical neurologic tests used to diagnose nerve injuries involve electromyography (EMG) and nerve conduction techniques that measure major motor or sensory nerve changes. A nerve conduction study (NCS)—also called a nerve conduction velocity (NCV) test—is a measurement of the speed of conduction of an electrical impulse through a nerve. NCS can determine nerve damage and destruction.

During the test, the nerve is stimulated, usually with surface electrode patches attached to the skin. Two electrodes are placed on the skin over the nerve. One electrode stimulates the nerve with a very mild electrical impulse and the other electrode records it. The resulting electrical activity is recorded by another electrode. This is repeated for each nerve being tested. The nerve conduction velocity (speed) is then calculated by measuring the distance between electrodes and the time it takes for electrical impulses to travel between electrodes.

A related procedure that may be performed is electromyography (EMG). An EMG measures the electrical activity in muscles and is often performed at the same time as NCS. Both procedures help to detect the presence, location, and extent of diseases that damage the nerves and muscles. A fine-needle electrode is inserted into the muscle tissue and electrical activity is studied. This procedure has been reported by my CRPS patients as especially painful. In my opinion, anything that involves insult to the sensory nervous system of a CRPS patient, such as a needle entering the body, should be avoided except for in life-threatening situations.

Unfortunately, the small-fiber nerve injuries in CRPS are not detected by these standard tools, which only measures large-fiber function. The difficulty in measuring small-fiber damage led one doctor (Dr. Oaklander) and her colleagues to propose skin biopsy for detection of CRPS.[41] Skin biopsy, a procedure in which a sample of skin tissue is removed and examined, provides a very sensitive method for detecting small nerve fiber damage. According to Dr. Oaklander, skin biopsies are actual windows into the peripheral nervous system, showing detailed changes associated with CRPS.

In her study, small skin samples were taken from eighteen adults with CRPS-I and seven people who had chronic pain from osteoarthritis, but not CRPS. Each subject identified the location of his or her maximum pain, a nearby symptom-free area on the same limb, and a pain-free area on the opposite limb. Skin biopsies were then taken from all three spots, and the density of tiny projections extending from each nerve cell (small nerve fibers, or neurites) was measured. The results showed a decrease in the number of neurites in the CRPS-affected regions only. On average, about 30 percent of the neurites were missing in the CRPS-affected limbs. It is further theorized that the loss of neurites may cause the pain of CRPS by triggering a hyperresponse on the part of the remaining neurons. This method is not yet in widespread use. In addition, there is the obvious drawback that removing a sample of skin from a CRPS patient is in and of itself an invasive procedure, which should always be avoided in CRPS cases when possible.

PHYSICAL EXAM

The value of a thorough physical exam by a doctor who knows what to look at cannot be overestimated. The typical CRPS patients will often give off physical clues that may seem small, but, in fact, may be crucial in obtaining the best diagnosis. A good exam starts with a thorough history taken by someone who really *listens* to the patient. Patients will report and demonstrate sensitivity to light touch, deep touch, pain, vibration, circumferential pressure, cold, heat, and increased pain when they experience bad weather. They will often report sensitivity to the touch of clothes, shoes, carpet underneath bare feet, showers, and so on. There are some clues that can be seen by visual observation alone, such as soft-tissue edema and enhancement, skin thickening, color changes, changes to the nails or hair, skin rashes and wounds and muscle atrophy in the later stages. In addition, patients who suffer from CRPS will show abnormalities of the III, VII, IX and X (parasympathetic) cranial nerves.

It is very difficult for any doctor when they are faced with a desperate patient, wanting an objective reason for why he or she is hurting. The current diagnostic tools are mere guides. The most important factor in every diagnosis is to get yourself to a doctor who is well familiar with the signs and symptoms of CRPS. A keen eye and experience cannot be recommended strongly enough when it comes to CRPS. If you have the smallest suspicion that your doctor is unfamiliar with CRPS and its presentation, you must fire that doctor immediately. Do not waste any time in obtaining a correct diagnosis. Time is very, very critical and not on your side.

I ran across the following quote on the rsdhope.org webpage that I found to be very true and wanted to share with you: *"Just because you can't find the exact source of someone's pain doesn't mean they don't feel it,"* says John F. Dombrowski, MD, a Washington, DC pain specialist. *"No test can measure the intensity of pain, no imaging device can show pain, and no instrument can locate pain precisely. This doesn't mean pain can't be treated. We don't need to know the exact cause of the pain to try to make it feel better."*

NAVIGATING THE CONFUSING MAZE OF TREATMENTS

Although I am known to be a big proponent of treating the cause rather than the symptom, and I try to teach my patients a mind-set that allows them to investigate and examine the root cause of their symptoms, CRPS has been humbling for me as a doctor. What I mean by this is that even the bravest patient cannot typically survive the sky-high pain levels that characterize CRPS without some kind of intervention or help from the outside. CRPS taught me that sometimes pain relief is not a luxury or a choice, but a necessity for simple survival. That being said, I have been humbled by the bravery I have encountered in many CRPS patients, who will refuse to reach for pain medication unless they are backed against a monstrous wall of pain. Because most CRPS patients have access to vast amounts of pain medications, this truly takes self-control. In this section, I will cover some of the treatments available to CRPS patients today. My list by no means can boast to be all-inclusive, but I will try my best to give you a good understanding of your options.

Please note that my opinion of any treatment is often based only upon my own research. It is not my intent to neither encourage nor discourage you from seeking a specific treatment. My only intent is to supply information in a fair and balanced manner. As with any treatment, you are responsible for researching any possible treatment that you may consider, including its pros and cons.

PAIN MEDICATION

The use of pain medication in the treatment of CRPS is common but somewhat controversial. In the United States especially, pain medications are usually used as the first line of defense when it comes to the treatment of CRPS. However, the successful treatment of CRPS is so elusive and looks very different in each patient, as no one seems to respond the same way. Very often, CRPS patients will tell me that they respond "differently than anyone else" when it comes to pain medications. I suspect that at least part of the reason for this is the MTHFR gene mutation that most CRPS patients seem to suffer from, as mentioned in chapter 4. Remember, this gene mutation will often cause your body to detoxify harmful substances, like medications, at a much slower than normal rate.

OPIOIDS

Opioids include medications such as morphine, hydromorphone, methadone, hydrocodone and oxycodone, and the fentanyl patch, to name a few. Considerable controversy exists regarding the use of opioids for treatment of chronic pain of noncancer origin, and this is especially true for CRPS. The most popular opinion is that opioids are not very effective in the treatment of chronic pain conditions of a neurologic nature. Currently, there are no well-controlled long-term studies showing long-term improvement in CRPS patients using opioids. However, many patients suffering from CRPS rely on opioids just to get through the day, and report that it does give them at least some pain relief. In my experience, when successful, opioids will typically lower the CRPS patients' pain about two points or so on the pain scale.

Side effects caused by the use of opioids are very common and may be dangerous. Common opioid side effects, particularly with higher doses, include constipation, dependency (not to be confused with addiction), nausea, vomiting, cognitive impairment, sleepiness, and trouble breathing. Longer the opioids are used, the higher the chances of experiencing side effects and addiction. In some cases, long-term use may even lead to something called hyperalgesia, meaning *increased* sensitivity to pain. Opioid use is very hard on your body, also. Both the liver and kidneys have to work overtime to rid your body of this class of drugs daily. Long-term use contributes to cellular toxicity, decreased immune function, and disruption of your hormones.

LYRICA

Lyrica was first approved for the use of fibromyalgia in 2007. Its side effects include weight gain, dizziness, drowsiness, dry mouth, speech disturbances, sinus infections, swelling of feet and hands, infections, headaches, double vision, accidental injury, and difficulty with concentration. In more serious cases, patients have reported severe allergic reactions to Lyrica, including hives, blisters, increased heart rate, itching, difficulty breathing, and swelling of the face and tongue. Lyrica may interact adversely to other medications, such as sleeping medications or some opioids, such as morphine. It is postulated that Lyrica actually addresses the symptoms of spinal cord pain rather than the indirect symptoms of CRPS. The EU (European Union) approved Lyrica for central spinal cord pain.

While Lyrica is certainly no magic bullet, most CRPS patients report that it relieves their pain at least moderately, although its success varies from patient to patient. Lyrica should never be stopped cold turkey. When my patients complete their treatment or enter the second phase of the intense part of their treatment, and report significant lower pain levels, I always refer them to a physician that can advise them about slowly tapering down their use of Lyrica.

CYMBALTA

Cymbalta is an antidepressant which is sometimes prescribed to treat nerve pain and other conditions off label. Similar to Lyrica, it is postulated that Cymbalta (duloxetine) actually addresses the symptoms of spinal cord pain rather than the indirect symptoms of CRPS. Side effects of Cymbalta include, but are not limited to: blindness, abdominal pain, blistering of skin, blurred vision, loss of consciousness, cold sweat, mental confusion, dark urine, decreased urine output, convulsions, impaired vision, difficulty swallowing, light-headedness when suddenly standing up, fainting, hives, loss of bladder control, uncontrollable jerking of extremities, shivering, sign of liver damage such as yellowing of the skin and sudden uncharacteristic feelings of excitement that you cannot control. Cymbalta should also be tapered down with the help of a physician. Most CRPS patients report a moderate level of pain relief using this medication. Cymbalta may interact with more than a thousand other drugs in a negative way (e.g., morphine), so make sure that your doctor checks the safety of *all* your drugs when taken together, not just individually.

LOW DOSE NALTREXONE (LDN)

In 1984 Naltrexone was approved by the FDA in a 50mg dose for helping heroin and opium addicts, by blocking the effect of these drugs, by blocking opioid receptors. . Naltrexone also blocks the reception of the opioid hormones that our brain and adrenal glands produce: beta-endorphin and metenkephalin. Many body tissues have receptors for these endorphins and enkephalins, including virtually every cell of the body's immune system.

In 1985, Bernard Bihari, MD, discovered the effects of a much smaller dose of naltrexone (approximately 3mg once a day) on the body's immune system. LDN is prescribed for a wide variety of conditions today, including cander, autoimmune conditions, and Central Nervous System disorders. It is believed to produce a prolonged up-regulation of vital elements of the immune system by causing an increase in endorphin and enkephalin production. LDN has shown great promise for lowering pain for some patients who suffer from CRPS. In addition, it is relatively inexpensive.

Commonly reported side effects of naltrexone include: streptococcal pharyngitis, fainting, anxiety, fatigue, drowsiness, nasopharyngitis, sedation, posttraumatic stress disorder, joint pain, headaches, panic attack, nausea, vomiting, pharyngitis, joint stiffness, nervousness, arthritis, dizziness, obsessive compulsive disorder, headache, sinus headache, stiffness, muscle spasm, muscle cramps, muscle rigidity, depression, and twitching. Less commonly, it may also cause depression, skin rashes, chest pain, ringing in the ears, and weight gain.

ALL THE OTHERS

There are many other drugs that are prescribed to CRPS patients. This list includes (but isn't limited to) Topamax (an antiseizure medication), Neurontin (or gabapentin, originally developed to treat epilepsy), NSAIDS, low-dose Naltrexone and many others. Please understand that of all the groups of chronic pain patients who have the right to reach out for pain medications, CRPS certainly should appear at the top of that list. I do urge you, however, to take every drug you decide to take under very careful consideration. You must never blindly trust any doctor (including myself) or pharmaceutical company, ever. It is *your* job to be your own advocate.

This means that you must carefully research every single drug you take in. Be aware of its potential side effects, negative interactions with other drugs as well as alcohol, and how to quit taking it, should that time arrive. You must also work hard to support your liver with detoxification (not to be done without help), a good diet, and supplementation, as described in chapter 12. Last but not least, never take a medication "just because." What do I mean by this? Astoundingly often, patients will tell me that they are taking something, even though they really can't tell if it is helping. If some time has gone by and you cannot tell a difference, why subject your body to this added chemical burden? *Only* take a medication if you can tell that there is a clear effective benefit while you are taking it.

CALMARE THERAPY

Calmare therapy disrupts the pain signal by "scrambling" it. It is suitable for severe, chronic, neuropathic and oncologic (cancer) pain patients exclusively using the MC5-A, a computerized medical device. This medical device has FDA clearance. The treatment incorporating this technology, called Scrambler Therapy (ST), uses disposable surface electrodes on the skin (similar but not the same as a TENS unit) to transmit synthetic nonpain information through surface nerve receptors. This treatment applies a low-amperage electric signal that is composed of codes recognized and normally used by the brain. These codes enter the body through dermatomes, (or specific areas of the skin known to be supplied by a single spinal root) to the dorsal (posterior) part of the spinal cord and central nervous system (CNS). The new code "tricks" the brain to read a discernable nonpain code as real and generated from itself. When this happens, there is a "zeroing out" of the pain. Through plasticity (the ability of the brain to adapt to change) the brain will then learn to expect, look for, and prefer the nonpain code.

This treatment is noninvasive, and should show results fairly soon, if it is going to work. It is typically paid for out of pocket as it is typically not covered by the insurance companies. Please note that this is often the case for successful more nontraditional treatments. You can find success stories all over the Internet about this therapy, and also CRPS patients for whom it did not work, unfortunately. Success is often determined by the severity of the case. It seems that patients with one limb respond better than patients in which the CRPS has spread. The one clear drawback appears to be that the treatment will often not last, and patients have to go back for additional treatments, which may be costly over time. Some patients report longer periods of relief and others only short periods.

If this treatment works exactly the way it claims to work, it will merely change the way the brain responds to pain, not the disruption in the CNS. If you do not address the nervous system dysfunction that gave rise to CRPS to begin with, you are still walking around with a ticking time bomb inside your body, which may give rise to other conditions or symptoms.

KETAMINE

Ketamine, discovered in 1962, is a medication mainly used for starting and maintaining anesthesia. Ketamine may be administered to CRPS patients in one of three methods—it may be used in a low-dose "awake" version, the "coma technique," or as an outpatient procedure. The "awake" version is the most widely used procedure today. The patient typically receives a dose of between 20 mg and 35 mg of ketamine, depending on several factors. The cost of this procedure varies between $10,000 and $50,000, and may be covered by insurance. It was pioneered by Dr. Correll, of Australia, and Dr. Ronald Harbut, of Hot Springs, Arkansas.

The "coma technique" is not FDA approved for use in the United States. The treatment used to be available in both Germany and Mexico, but the German program was shut down, reportedly after at least one patient passed away after undergoing this procedure. During this procedure, the patient is placed in a deep five-day coma, during which they have to be placed on a ventilator. The procedure has almost the same effect on the CNS as hitting "Control," "Alt" and "Delete" on your computer keyboard. It reboots the CNS, often resulting in the pain to massively decrease or disappear, sometimes for long periods of time. The cost of this procedure is in excess of $60,000. The outpatient procedure is not reported to be very effective at all.

One article sums up the way ketamine works in the following manner: "Although Ketamine may have more than one mechanism of action, the basis for using it to treat RSD/CRPS may reside in its strong ability to block NMDA receptors. Experimental evidence suggests that a sufficiently intense or prolonged painful stimulus causes an extraordinary release of glutamate from peripheral nociceptive afferents onto dorsal horn neurons within the spinal cord. The glutamate released, in turn, stimulates NMDA receptors on second-order neurons that produce the phenomena of windup and central sensitization. It is reasonable to consider that, by blocking NMDA receptors, one might also be able to block cellular mechanisms supporting windup and central sensitization. Ketamine is the only potent NMDA-blocking drug currently available for clinical use. Our interpretation is that an appropriately prolonged infusion of Ketamine appears to maintain a level of Ketamine in the central nervous system long enough to reverse the effects of the sensitization process and associated pain."[42]

NMDA (N-methyl-D-aspartate) receptor is a glutamate receptor and ion channel protein found in the nerve cells. Glutamate is a nerve cell messenger that causes excitation (excitement) in the nerve cells. It may cause harm when its messages become overwhelming. You may say that NMDA is the lock, and glutamate is the key. When the key unlocks the lock it causes excitement in the nerve cells. If this process becomes ongoing, it may cause chronic pain.

Ketamine is known as one of the most effective treatments for CRPS today. However, all that means is that it is more effective than most other treatments for longer periods of time. Although ketamine has been known to cause remission in some lucky patients, most patients seem to have to go back repeatedly for expensive booster treatments. In addition, ketamine may have quite severe side effects, even permanent neurologic injury or death in the case of the coma treatment. It has been shown that ketamine has negative stimulatory effects on cardiac function and is related to the systemic release of catecholamines (their release by sympathetic nerve endings increases the rate and force of muscular contraction of the heart), *inhibition* of the vagal nerve (the very thing that contributes to CRPS to begin with), and inhibition of norepinephrine reuptake at peripheral nerves and nonneuronal tissues such as the myocardium. Heart muscle depression has been observed after high-dose ketamine infusions or during repeated dosing.

It is my hypothesis that ketamine changes the nervous system for often long periods of time, if not permanently. No study that I could find has ever been performed to study the long-term changes of ketamine in the human body. It is my experience that for my treatment, ketamine represents somewhat of a "wild card" effect, in that it will sometimes make the patient not respond to treatment as well as other CRPS patients, especially if the ketamine treatments have been recent.

Again, ketamine does not address the original *cause* of CRPS, but rather changes the nervous system.

SPINAL-CORD STIMULATORS

Approved by the FDA in 1989, spinal cord stimulation (SCS) has become a common treatment for patients with chronic pain in their back or limbs, who have not found pain relief from other treatments. Soft, thin wires with electrical leads on their tips are placed through a needle in the back near to the spinal column. The leads are placed through a needle inserted in the back (no incision is required). A small incision is then made and a tiny, programmable generator is placed under the skin. There it emits electrical currents to the spinal column.

Some CRPS patients report a significant decrease in daily pain after getting a SCS. Others report no relief or even an increase in pain after the procedure. For some, it may work for a while and then stop being as effective. As with any implanted device, infection can occur. The lead, extension, or neurostimulator could move within the body or push through the skin. There could be undesirable changes in stimulation. It is also possible that the implanted materials (as with any foreign object in the body) may cause an allergic or immune system response. The device might unexpectedly cease to function due to battery depletion or other causes.

Another side effect of SCS is that it may cause scarring. Scar tissue can be very detrimental to the health of your nervous system. Nerve communication moves through cells in a wavelike pattern, rather than electricity moving through a wire. In fact, electricity in a nerve is not like an electric current at all. An electric current is a rapid flow of electrons, but electricity sweeps along the nerve as an "action potential," a difference in electrical charge between the outside and the inside of the nerve.[43] Think of a wave moving through water. If there is a rock in that body of water, the rock will cause a "break" in the wave pattern. Much like the rock, the nerve "wave" cannot move through the scar tissue like it moves through the healthy tissue. This will often result in an increase in pain and resistance to successful treatment. In addition, it is an invasive procedure which is always risky when treating CRPS. The cost of a SCS is usually more than $50,000 with significant annual upkeep. However, insurance companies will often cover it. Spinal cord stimulators are not FDA approved for the treatment of CRPS.

PAIN (DRUG) PUMPS

Drug pumps, or intrathecal drug delivery devices, deliver pain medication directly to the fluid-filled area surrounding the spinal cord (called the intrathecal space). The system consists of a pump and catheter (a thin, flexible tube), both of which are surgically implanted under the skin. The pump is a round device that stores and delivers pain medication, and is typically implanted in your abdomen. The catheter is placed in a small space created by the surgeon at the spine and connected to the pump. With this system, pain medication goes directly to the pain receptors near the spine, instead of going through the circulatory system. For that reason, drug pumps offer significant pain control using just a fraction of the dose that oral medication requires.

Since this procedure requires surgery, complications (made more possible by the presence of CRPS) or infection may occur. Once implanted, several complications may occur with the device, such as the catheter leaking or tearing, or becoming disconnected. The pump or catheter may move or wear through the skin. These complications may require surgery. The pump may stop if the battery runs out. Drug overdose or underdose can result in serious complications and may even be life-threatening. The typical side effects of the drug being delivered should also be considered. The formation of an inflammatory mass at the tip of catheter has been reported, which may lead to serious complications, such as paralysis. The same problems with scarring that occurs with spinal cord stimulators may occur with drug pumps. In my experience, at least external scarring is rather significant in most patients. The body does not like foreign objects inside of it, and will often react to it in various adverse ways.

SYMPATHECTOMY

Sympathectomy is performed to interrupt the portion of the patient's sympathetic nervous system (SNS) that is affected by CRPS. During sympathectomy, the sympathetic ganglia that cause CRPS pain are cut surgically, or chemically destroyed. It may also be destroyed with radiofrequency. Surgical sympathectomies are irreversible procedures. Sympathetic ganglia are collections of nerve cells that occur in clusters along the mid or lower spinal cord. It is especially recommended for patients who have received significant pain relief from sympathetic nerve blocks. Sympathetic nerve blocks involve injecting anesthetics into sympathetic nerves that are affected by CRPS. Sympathectomies are extremely controversial, as there is little evidence to fully support the efficacy of the procedure. Many doctors (including myself) deem this procedure risky due to the irreversible damage to sympathetic nerves.

This procedure causes nerve signals to be irreparably disrupted. These signals would normally travel to many different organs, glands, and muscles. Sympathectomies will distort many bodily functions, including vascular responses, sweating, heart rate, thyroid function, pupil dilation, lung volume, skin temperature, and the vitally important fight-or-flight response. It also reduces the physiological responses to strong emotions, such as fear, alertness, arousal, and laughter. In addition, it has been shown that it may cause immune system dysfunction, as well as acquired cardiovascular disease. Chemical sympathectomies may lead to sympathetic sprouting, as described in chapter 6. This may cause the pain of CRPS to return even more intensely than before. Sympathectomies are typically "last resort" procedures for patients who face edema, tissue loss, and recurrent infection.

TRANSCRANIAL MAGNETIC STIMULATION

TMS is a noninvasive method used to stimulate small, specific regions of the brain. A magnetic field generator, or "coil," is placed near the head of the person receiving the treatment during a TMS procedure. The coil produces small electric currents in the region of the brain just under the coil. The coil is connected to a pulse generator, or stimulator, that delivers an electric current to the coil. It is hypothesized that TMS affects the central nervous system much the same as ketamine does, but without all the nasty side effects. Unfortunately, while TMS does seem to provide some relief for patients, it does not seem to work for everyone, and most often does not seem permanent. Some within the CRPS community have questioned whether the level and durations of relief warrant the cost involved (about $10,000 for a series, although some clinics may charge less). TMS is FDAl approved for migraines and major depression only, and not all insurance companies will cover this treatment.

The greatest risks of TMS are the rare occurrence of fainting and even less commonly, seizures, also not very common. Other unwanted effects of TMS include discomfort or pain, transient induction of a mild form of mania, transient cognitive changes (that interferes with your thinking), temporary hearing loss, and impairment of working memory. It may cause problems with pacemakers.

NERIDRONATE

In 2014, the FDA finally acknowledged that CRPS is indeed, a rare condition. This has vast implications for pharmaceutical companies, as this is a game changer when it comes to CRPS research. These companies may now receive attractive tax breaks, and may include fewer subjects in any studies necessary to prove the efficacy of a drug developed specifically for CRPS. In addition, such companies may market the drug for seven years without threat of competition. This is getting a lot of corporate attention. The first company to launch such research in the United States was Grunenthal, a German-based company, and the trial medication is neridronate, also known as amino-bisphosphonate. This study is expected to be completed in 2016.

Significant attention has been focused on this drug, since a very small but successful trial was completed in Italy.[44] The inclusion for this trial was very strict, as no one whose CRPS onset was greater than four months ago was allowed to participate. This study reported a good outcome of up to a year. Surprisingly, the placebo group in this study also reported a marked initial decrease in pain. The US study trial's inclusion will not be as strict, with the exception of patients who suffer from CRPS Type 2, meaning that nerve damage can be detected. Neridronate has been used in Europe for quite some time now. Bisphosphonates are a class of drugs that prevent the loss of bone mass and are used to treat osteoporosis and similar diseases. Bone undergoes constant transformation and is kept in balance by specific bone cells called osteoblasts (that create bone) and osteoclasts (that destroy bone). Bisphosphonates inhibit the destruction of bone by encouraging osteoclasts to undergo cell death, thereby slowing bone loss. It does not encourage new bone growth, but it simply slows down bone loss.

The side effects of this drug include muscle tremors, muscle and joint pain, inflammation of the eye, fever, cardiac arrhythmia, atrial fibrillation, thyroid problems,[45] and jaw necrosis[46]. Since this last side effect is often glossed over, I want to make sure that we address it in detail so that you understand the gravity of it. Necrosis means *dying* of the bones that form the jaw and house the teeth. This is not an uncommon side effect at all. This occurs more often when bisphosphonates are administered through IV, rather than orally. One large study found that 20 percent of IV bisphosphonate users will develop necrosis of the jaw. There is no way to prevent this side effect. It is most often triggered by dental work after the drug has been administered, especially any kind of dental surgery. The risk remains high for the lifetime of the patient. Many dentists will not agree to work on a patient who has taken this drug, due to fear of complications. The symptoms of jaw necrosis include bad breath, lock jaw, abscesses, pockets of pus, loosening teeth, numbness in the face, feeling of heaviness in the jaw, and swelling of the gums or face.

Much hope is being focused on the current US trial. Caution is advised, however, since the safety of taking this drug long term has not been studied, and the known side effects are potentially serious. There is no word yet on possible insurance coverage of this treatment nor the cost of this treatment.

HYPERBARIC CHAMBERS

Hyperbaric oxygen therapy (HBOT) is a form of treatment that is recommended for many different types of diseases and ailments. The most recognized use of HBOT is to help scuba divers recover from "the bends," or decompression sickness. HBOT works as a treatment for CRPS by saturating all body tissues with oxygen. This first relieves any oxygen deprivation that has come from the swelling or tissue damage. It may also relieve swelling and increase circulation. Possible symptoms or side effects after HBOT can include fatigue, light-headedness, lung damage, sinus damage, changes in vision (nearsightedness), lung failure, seizures, and fluid buildup in the lungs. Side effects are generally mild as long as the therapy lasts no longer than two hours and the pressure inside the chamber is less than three times that of the normal pressure in the atmosphere.

There are currently about fourteen ailments that the FDA has approved HBOT as a treatment for, but CRPS is not one of them. For this reason, insurance companies will often not cover HBOT. The typical treatment series for CRPS is about forty sessions with additional treatments after as needed. Treatment cost is typically about $250–$300 per session. HBOT is noninvasive and typically won't make patients worse. CRPS patients report varying degrees of success with this treatment, although many find it beneficial. One drawback is that the patient cannot always tell early on if HBOT will work for them, which can make it a costly trial.

MARIJUANA

Few subjects (other than politics or religion) are as polarizing as the medical use of marijuana (*Cannabis*) for pain, even within the CRPS community, where people understand chronic pain better than most. However, writing a book about CRPS and not discussing marijuana news will reflect poorly on me as its author. That being said, I want to make it clear that I am not firmly in either camp regarding this subject. I see both plusses and minuses on both sides. If you live in a state where the use of marijuana is illegal, I am obviously not advising you to start using it.

As we all know, the use of medical marijuana has been approved by only a few states in the United States, although the movement to legalize it is gaining more steam, and the issue is slowly making it onto more ballots countrywide. Worldwide, it is illegal in most countries although some countries have decriminalized it, which basically means that these counties consider it a "soft" drug and have turned a blind eye to its usage (the Netherlands, for instance).

At least one study has shown a positive effect on sleep as well as pain with moderate daily *Cannabis* usage.[47] However, even this study cautioned that the long-term effects of marijuana, as well as any addictive components, have not been studied yet. Although the smoke from burning marijuana flowers contains several cancer-causing compounds, similar to those found in tobacco smoke, smoking marijuana has been shown to be vastly less damaging to the lungs than tobacco by at least one very large-scale study.[48] It is thought that the reason for this is that the smoke from marijuana contains several unique compounds called cannabinoids (e.g., THC and CBD) which have been shown to have significant anticancer and antitumor effects. Nevertheless, smoking marijuana may still be irritating to the lungs, causing conditions like bronchitis and asthma. For this reason, vaporizers are recommended for most people using it for medicinal purposes. Vaporizers greatly reduce the risk of airway irritation.

No matter how marijuana enters your body, it affects almost every organ in your body, as well as your nervous system and immune system. Smoking pot can increase your heart rate by as much as two times for up to three hours. Other effects include feeling "high," red eyes and dilated pupils, increased appetite, slowed reaction time (making it dangerous to drive), dry mouth, dizziness, shallow breathing, feelings of paranoia, anxiety, depression, short-term memory loss, and an ongoing cough.

Marijuana can be addictive for some people. Even if you buy marijuana from a legal, state regulated dispensary, it is impossible to know with 100 percent certainty how much THC it contains, making its effects and potential for addiction hard to predict. If you are male, marijuana can lower your libido, sperm count and quality. It has been shown by some research that there is a link between marijuana use and some mental health problems, such as depression and suicidal thoughts, although this research remains controversial. Unfortunately, very few truly objective parties choose to study the effects of long-term marijuana use, which greatly impacts the study outcomes, in my opinion. The long-term effects of possible toxicity in the brain has not been studied adequately.

The human body is designed to function a certain way without outside interference. Besides good nutrition and water, as well as sunshine and oxygen, it really requires little to self-regulate. We were not designed to inhale a substance every day, ingesting chemicals that alter the way our minds work and our bodies function every day. However, it is hard to come by a better reason to do so than suffering from the pain of CRPS every day. In addition, it is much less harmful than the drugs CRPS patients take to control pain every day. In my opinion, you should be honest and mindful about your daily usage. Some people fall in the habit of getting high first thing in the morning, every day. Gauge your usage while using your pain as a guide. Use it as needed, and not just because it becomes a way of life. Treat it with the same respect that you treat any other chemical that enters your body.

Next, let's delve into the system that we use in our clinic.

10

A New Way: Healing the Central Nervous System

The master maker of the human body did not create you and then run off and leave you masterless.

—B. J. Palmer

Old ways don't open new doors.

—T. Mac

I often find myself talking to other physicians across the globe, and invariably, they ask me the same question: "Why RSD/CRPS? Why in the world would you choose to specialize in such a difficult condition?" I always answer the same way: "How could I not?" I have always maintained that CRPS picked me, I didn't pick it. Ever since I treated my very first patient suffering from CRPS, I became obsessed with helping people who suffers from this horrible, life-robbing condition. I hunted down doctors and techniques from all over the world, determined to figure out how to help the body beat this condition. If I heard that someone was having success treating CRPS, I wanted to know what they knew. I had two rules that I held sacred while studying other treatment methods: all treatments had to involve healing the central nervous system, and no treatment could possibly harm the patient in any way. Along the way, I got to witness some incredible recoveries. I was amazed at the results my staff and I were getting, yet frustrated that very few knew about it. I soon realized that another book was in my future. I could not sit on the information I now had in my hands without sharing it.

While researching my book, I realized that CRPS has touched many other doctors in a similar way. You cannot treat this condition and witness the path of destruction that it cuts across people's lives, without becoming singularly obsessed with helping people who suffer from it recover. I am hardly the first physician to ever develop a passion to beat this thing. Early on my new path, a doctor once told me that seeing miracles, and being part of those miracles, is a very addictive thing. I can only agree with that statement wholeheartedly.

WHAT MAKES OUR TREATMENT DIFFERENT?

While learning how to treat the neurologic symptoms of CRPS, my basic holistic training and upbringing have come in very handy. That training has taught me that, unlike the mechanistic approach (that which most medical doctors follow today), the body is *not* like an engine. What I mean by that is that you cannot just treat different parts, forgetting that every part is connected to every other part. The body is incredibly intelligent, far above our understanding as human beings. Just think about all the trillions of functions happening in your body every second of every day—things we cannot even comprehend. Your immune system is fighting off invaders and cancer cells every day. Trillions of cells are being repaired or replaced; hormones are being produced; vitamins are being gathered from the food you eat and delivered to the cells that need them. All of this without a second thought from you.

We readily expect our body to do these incredible things every day. Yet, we just accept that somehow our bodies become broken beyond repair, not smart enough to beat "incurable" conditions. We accept that this power now rests in the doctors' hands, and that we will find "magic" in some form of surgery, device or medication. Something outside of yourself. Especially when fear hits.

Putting Out the Fire

All the scientists in the world cannot even grow a hair. Yet, our body does that every day. The intelligence that runs this all day doesn't just desert some of us one day, causing us to suffer. So, how do we get sick then? Something interferes with the way our bodies are supposed to run and heal from the inside out. In my experience, and always in the case of CRPS, this interference typically happens in the central nervous system.

Together with our treatment system, we believe that there is one crucial ingredient that should be part of patient care. I call this, our "secret sauce."

THE SECRET SAUCE

When I first wrote an outline for this chapter, I thought I would end with this topic. After giving it some thought, however, I have decided that it should come first. It is probably *the* most important part of our treatment. When I went to chiropractic school, the legendary founder of that school (Parker College of Chiropractic), Dr. Jim Parker, was also the president. He was a little guy with a huge personality. He regularly smoked cigars breezing right by the "no smoking" signs through the hallways at Parker. He had a *huge* personality and hugged everyone he met, often random students. He taught me one of the most important concepts I would ever learn when it comes to patient care, which he called "The love concept." What this entailed was simple: truly caring about your patients. When you love the patient, obstacles to healing disappear and symptoms tend to get better. Your patient *knows* when you truly care and when you do not.

I have been told through the years that a doctor should not become attached to their patient. I have come to accept that whether prudent or not, I *am* attached to my patients. I am incredibly invested in each patient. I feel that it is a tremendous privilege for a patient to trust me enough to let me work on their body.

I learn about my patients' families and their struggles and their hopes and dreams. I cry with them and I celebrate with them, and when I cannot help them, it makes me lie awake at night, questioning what I could have done better, how I can keep from failing next time.

This love carries over into our practice. I tend to hire staff members that have once been sick themselves. They are most often former patients of mine. They have to understand our patients' pain, as this makes them more sympathetic and truly caring. Our practice has a friendly family atmosphere, and there is much socializing among our patients. We encourage the support that patients can give each other. When you call our phone, I often pick up myself. It tends to throw patients. "You mean you are the *doctor?*" Yes, I am the doctor, and it is important that we connect if I am to help you or your family member. I am not too important or too busy to pick up a phone. When you go through treatment, you work with me every day, not a PA, CA, or some other stand-in. When you tell me your history, I am the one to write it down. I am the one heading your treatment, and I should be the one who understands every aspect of your health and how you got sick.

> *I will remember that there is art to medicine as well as science, and that warmth, sympathy, and understanding may outweigh the surgeon's knife or the chemist's drug. I will not be ashamed to say "I know not," nor will I fail to call in my colleagues when the skills of another are needed for a patient's recovery.*
>
> —Hippocratic oath

You need a doctor who, above all else, truly cares about you. Doctors are not gods. They are not power figures who may not be questioned. We work for *you*. Like any good employee, if we are to help you, we have to listen to you and care about you. I throw my passion into every single case that I treat. Every patient represents a goal to me. When listening to my patients, I don't just want to hear about their pain; I want to know what CRPS took away from them. What is it that they miss? Is it to walk their beloved dog? To travel with their husband? To work in the job they love? To enjoy their grandchildren? These are the things I want them to get back.

This is the reason I have a fire burning in my heart, and passion filling my days. It is not just about beating the monster...it's about being charged and blessed with the responsibility to help guide people just like you back to *life*, instead of merely surviving and living "around" your pain. You deserve to live with passion again. You deserve to be happy. You deserve to be *alive* again with joy.

The other side of the coin is what the patient brings to the table. Every patient I have ever watched recover had one thing in common—*spirit*. It takes tremendous courage to keep looking for ways to recover, regardless of how many times you have been disappointed in the past. It takes grit! I often find myself across from a new patient, holding their two-inch thick medical file, filled with medical records. Each one of those records represents a time when you sat across from a doctor, looking for answers, looking for help, hoping that *this* time will give you back your life again. My heart goes out to you, it truly does. Yet, you cannot give up. You cannot stop looking for ways to aid your body in recovering, no matter how many times you have been disappointed.

Now, let's look at exactly what you can expect when you come to our clinic for treatment.

EXPOSING THE MAKINGS OF A MONSTER: TESTING

When a patient enters our clinic, our first task is to examine the central nervous system thoroughly. While the average patient suffering from CRPS has often seen neurologists before, and have undergone countless tests, such as X-rays, MRIs, and nerve conduction tests, our tests (and how they are interpreted) are all designed to detect one thing: nerve interference, affecting the body on a global scale, allowing it to malfunction and often causing excruciating unrelenting daily pain. None of our tests are painful or invasive. I strongly feel that it is important to always remember when it comes to patients suffering from CRPS to first, to first do no harm.

We do not do a single test that will not also help us to treat you. One of my pet peeves is inappropriate, expensive, and unnecessary diagnostic testing. A test should be taken for one reason only—in order to understand the patient's body better, so that you can treat them in the most effective way possibly, or refer them somewhere else.

SURFACE ELECTROMYOGRAPHY EXAM (SEMG)

The central nervous system consists of the brain and spinal cord. Think of the spinal cord as the highway that connects the brain to the body. If the exits of this highway are blocked, that will lead to cars piling up and not getting to go to their destination. Nerve signals coming from and to the brain can be blocked in the same way, affecting how well the body is able to function and heal. The EMG scan is a reliable method[49–51] to measure changes in the electrical activity of paraspinal muscles. Changes in paraspinal muscle function are seen in vertebral subluxation (or abnormalities). Taken in concert with other examination findings, EMG scans are useful in detecting and characterizing the muscular dysfunction seen in vertebral abnormalities affecting the central nervous system.

This test is done by wetting the skin of your back with alcohol and then gently placing electrodes on each side of the spine at each vertebral level. In a good candidate for treatment, we expect to see abnormalities especially in the upper cervical and lower lumbar spine.

HEART RATE VARIABILITY (HRV) EXAM

HRV is the variation in the length of time between one heartbeat and the next. Most people think that ideally, this space should be exactly the same every time but in fact, the opposite is true. You want it to constantly change. We generally think of a number between 60 and 90 when we think of our heart rate. Your heart rate changes all the time. For example, when you inhale your heart rate speeds up and when you exhale it slows down. So the heart rate will actually vary between, say, 70 and 80. HRV is a measure of this naturally occurring differences in your heart rate. Heart rate variability is a great indicator of vagus nerve function.[52]

HRV is almost like a crystal ball that allows us to gain insight into the health of the nervous system. It has been shown that people who suffer from CRPS have an increased heart rate and decreased heart rate variability. These findings were consistent with a general autonomic imbalance in those patients.[53] In fact, the activity of the vagus nerve as measured by HRV has been shown by studies to reveal all sorts of crucial data. For example, it has been shown, after studying patients suffering from late-stage cancer, the patients with higher vagus nerve activity has substantially lower levels of tumor markers in their systems when compared to patients with lower vagus nerve activity.[54] In addition, HRV allows us to determine how much functional reserve the patient has. Functional reserve could be likened to a "savings account" in your body. It's what your body has in reserve to help in times of need from illness, injury, and stress. HRV can also give us information regarding the nerve communication to the neurohormonal system, the immune system, the digestive system, the cardiac system, longevity, and can even predict whether someone is a good athlete.

HRV is noninvasive and does not hurt. It does not involve needles or any other invasive procedures.

FULL-SPINE X-RAYS

When indicated, we will take a full-spine X-ray series of your spine. When we study your X-rays, we are very interested in the health of your spine as this directly relates to the health of your central nervous system. An unhealthy spine points to poor nerve communication in the body. In addition to degeneration, arthritis and pathologies, we also check for form and function. We are especially interested in the upper cervical spine as well as the lower lumbar spine.

META-OXY INFLAMMATION TEST

This test is a simple urine test that measures inflammation in the body by showing us how much cell membrane damage is occurring in your body by free radicals. The outer protective shell that holds the cell together is critical. It's literally where all the communication takes place. The membrane basically functions as the brain of the cell. It is vital in communication, as signals from our nervous system, immune system, endocrine system, and other systems in the body attach to this membrane and tell the cells what to do. Failure to do so may cause damaged DNA, poor hormone regulation, accelerated aging, poor healing, heart problems, increased toxicity, and many other unwanted things or conditions.

HEAVY-METAL URINE TEST

We utilize a urine test to test for heavy-metal toxicity, as the hair analysis test is known to show unreliable results and poor reference ranges.[55] The urine test shows what metals are currently circulating in the body and being excreted by the kidney. It is a good indicator of chronic heavy-metal exposure.

After we complete our tests, we proceed with the treatment. Our hope is that every patient will leave the treatment and return to *life*, as opposed to merely surviving.

THE FOUR-PUNCH SYSTEM

Often, I am asked why there are not more doctors that do what we do. The answer is that we do not just use one specific therapy or approach. Our treatment is composed of a system that I have developed over many years, based on different treatment modalities and many years of experience. Think of it as a cookie recipe, where you add different ingredients together. If you isolate only one ingredient, you may get some results, but probably not optimum results. The chocolate chips are good but they do not quite taste the same as the whole cookie.

The trickiest part of our treatment is figuring out what each patient needs. In my experience, every single patient is different and must be approached differently. Treating the nervous system of someone who suffers from CRPS is agonizingly tricky sometimes. In some cases one treatment works better than others, and sometimes you have to combine more than one treatment at the same time, rather than splitting them up. Some patients respond within a minute each time, and others take longer. Nevertheless, I have a system that can be tweaked to fit each patient's needs. I have lovingly dubbed our approach as the "Three Punch System," as in, three punches and you are out. Recently, we had to revise it as the "Four Punch System," as we added a new treatment.

Typically, we recommend that the patient comes for a "testing period" of one to two weeks. During this time-period, we perform tests and start treating the patient with our system if appropriate. In order to continue care, we must see dramatic results during this initial testing period, or we do not proceed with care. Our treatment program lasts ten weeks on average (although it could be shorter) and typically, we recommend some follow-up care with a local doctor near the patient that we work with, or homecare, depending on every unique case. Most of our patients travel long distances to visit us, so we have to tailor their maintenance care depending upon their locations. While many of our patients who report full remission have not followed through with this maintenance care, I still get nervous when a patient decides to "fly solo" after the care. It is my job to make sure that we do everything in our power to make sure that your results are stable long term. My local patients usually remain under my care for some maintenance.

FIRST PUNCH: WAKING UP THE VAGUS NERVE

As discussed in chapter 6, the vagus nerve runs anterior to the highest cervical vertebra, called the atlas inside a structure called the carotid sheath. When the atlas is misplaced or misaligned, it can put pressure on the vagus nerve by pulling on it or pushing on it. More doctors are discovering that if you can wake up the vagus nerve, amazing things start to happen in the body, and inflammation is sometimes instantly switched off, resulting in a dramatic decrease in pain. The methods of doing this vary. Early research shows that is possible to implant a device (much like a pacemaker) that mechanically is stimulated with a magnet by the patient a few times a day that will "reboot" the vagus nerve. Other doctors use surgery, where sometimes part of the vertebra is removed, or a balloon placed in the jugular vein and inflated, in order to put pressure on the vagus nerve.

As with everything I do, I believe that if something can be done without creating more trauma to the body, this is vastly preferable.

The technique that I use to accomplish this was first developed to treat fibromyalgia. Over time, it became apparent that people who suffer from CRPS also responded to it very well. Before a patient enters treatment with this upper cervical technique, the patient is tested first to see if they are a good candidate for treatment. This test consists of gentle pressure applied in specific combinations to the upper cervical spine. If the patient has the neurological symptoms associated with some cases of CRPS caused by cervical trauma or stenosis, their pain will most often notably and dramatically decrease (although temporarily) while this pressure is applied. This lets me know that the patient will most likely respond favorably to care. Please note that the patient's response to this test cannot be predicted by failure to obtain results through previous chiropractic adjustments. In other words, even if chiropractic didn't work for you in the past, you may still respond to this one specific technique.

The technique is fantastic as the test lets us know immediately if the chance of success is likely. While there are no guarantees, and I do not possess a crystal ball, I have two great fears that tend to haunt me and shape the way I screen patients for care. My first fear is that I will treat a patient and ultimately not help them. My second fear is that I can help a patient, but for some reason, do not realize that early and give up too soon. Therefore, we do everything in our power to make sure that these two things do not happen in our clinic. The initial testing period helps to increase our chance of success.

The treatment itself consists of a series of specific adjustments to the upper cervical spine over a certain prescribed period of time. In order to accomplish this, we use a tool that gently moves the atlas back where it belongs. This tool is a spring-loaded, hand-held mechanical instrument that provides a quick, low-force impulse (sometimes with a torque if needed) at specific points. This procedure has to be repeated very often over a predetermined treatment period. This is because the ligaments in your upper cervical spine may be used to the old "wrong" position. There may also be scarring in the spine or soft tissues. All of these structures have to become used to their new corrected position. Think of the braces on your teeth. It won't work if you only wear it for one day.

The theory is that this tool is highly effective because of two distinct reasons: the first is based on the speed of the device. The instrument is so quick that the body's muscles are less likely to tense in response, and resist the treatment, as patients are sometimes apt to do, especially if they are in a lot of pain. The lack of muscle resistance may facilitate the treatment effectiveness. The second is that the applied force is localized and specific and does not add any bending movement to the joint.

While ongoing research is still needed, it is also theorized that this treatment decreases meningeal compression. The meninges are three layers that surround the brain and spinal cord and can become trapped, pulled, or compressed after neck or head trauma. This technique causes a massive normalizing shift of the autonomic or automatic nervous system. This often results in the patient feeling almost euphoric and very relaxed during and immediately after the test. I have made a dramatic difference in many patients' lives using this work as one of my tools, and I highly recommend it if you are suffering from not only CRPS, but any chronic pain condition such as fibromyalgia, migraines, failed surgeries, POTS, and many others.

It is important that you know that this technique does not hurt. It is very gentle and in most cases, may be used even after a patient has suffered from significant neck trauma or even after surgeries or spinal cord injuries.

SECOND PUNCH: FREQUENCY SPECIFIC MICROCURRENT (FSM)

In order to stimulate and encourage healing of the tissues, we use FSM. There is much to be done in this department if a patient suffers from CRPS. The inflammation needs to be decreased all the way from the spinal cord to the nerves. We must remove scar tissue, and help the body to heal ligaments, muscles, bones, and nerves. In addition, we need to stop the nerves from "leaking" sodium, potassium, and calcium. FSM is used to accomplish all this.

What is Microcurrent? It is a *very* small current (millionths of an ampere), too small to be detected by the sensory nerves. An ampere is a measure of the movement of electrons past a certain point, and it tells us how strong an electric current is. Because the current is so small, it is not painful, even for CRPS patients. It is the same kind of current your body naturally produces in each cell. It is also FDA approved. Microcurrent was first used by doctors in Europe about three decades ago to stimulate acupressure points and stimulating bone repair in fractures that would not heal.

At least one study has shown that microcurrent increased ATP production in rat skin 500 percent. ATP is the chemical that the body uses for energy in order to perform all its functions, including healing. The current also increased amino acid transport into the cells by 70 percent, as well as waste product removal.[56] Obviously, this will greatly encourage repair and healing in tissues.

When we look at cells at a subatomic (smaller than the atom) level, we realize that cells are made up of tiny particles called protons, electrons, and neutrons. These particles continuously move around (vibrate). Every specific tissue has a frequency that is unique to that tissue, like a fingerprint or a signature. FSM utilizes to channels that deliver the current to the body. One addresses a specific tissue by targeting its frequency, and the other neutralizes a specific condition or pathology. Again, the current is too small to be perceived by the patient and does not hurt.

There are no known negative side effects or risks to the patient, although the patient may experience a brief detoxification reaction after initial treatments. We therefore encourage patients to drink a lot of water both prior to and after treatments. Not only does it minimize detoxification, but it also increases the success of the treatment (as you know water is a great conductor of electricity).

FSM is taught by Carolyn McMakin, DC, one of my favorite mentors. She and George Douglas, DC, developed a system whereby we use specific frequencies clinically, using the FSM device, effective in treating different conditions, including the neurologic dysfunction that often results in CRPS. Doctor McMakin used this system to treat her own son's nervous system. He suffered from CRPS. As a result, his body healed his CRPS after his central nervous system was normalized using FSM. When combined with our two other systems, we find that this treatment is an incredibly effective part of the treatment of the neurologic symptoms of CRPS.

THIRD PUNCH: REHABILITATING THE NERVOUS SYSTEM

Lastly, we use a system called Quantum Neurology, developed by Dr. George Gonzalez, DC. This system was designed to rehabilitate every aspect of the nervous system. Dr. Gonzalez developed this system in order to treat his wife, Lori, after she suffered a spinal cord injury. After seeing countless famous doctors all over the country, Dr. Gonzalez realized that no single system existed that was designed to rehabilitate the nervous system. His work was based upon the premise that if the body suffers from a chronic injury, the brain will eventually start "ignoring" this injury. The reason for this is that the injury will act as an "energy vampire," robbing the rest of the body of energy on a daily basis in order to rush the stolen energy to the sight of the chronic injury, much like a slow "energy leak." As you know, energy cannot be created or destroyed. However, it can be transferred. Now, let's pretend that we can put a monetary value on energy, and your body is allowed $100 in order to survive every day. Every function will require some money. For example, walking may require $5 per leg, digestion $3, and so on. If you have a chronic injury (such as CRPS) the body will start to ignore it, or else the injury will rob all the other functions and body parts of their share of this $100. This will cause the body to function at less than optimum. This is a necessary function, but it does not encourage healing of chronic injuries when we need it.

When you take a painkiller, the body will have to rob its other functions and parts of valuable energy to devote to eliminating the painkiller.

As a result, the body stops paying attention to the injury (like a whimpering baby), in order to pay attention to the *screaming* baby, the toxic chemical that is the painkiller. As a result, you no longer feel the pain, and this brings relief. In much the same way, injuries that are being ignored because they result in "energy leaking" are not being worked on, and they are being ignored. When you suffer from CRPS, this is not a good thing, obviously. The monster that is CRPS is being treated by the body as a whimpering baby, instead of a screaming one.

In order to heal glitches in the nervous system, we must first "show" the brain (or remind it) that the nervous system is injured, and then assist the brain in healing the injury. We use this system to very gently heal the abnormal sensory nerves (which are causing you to be in pain when exposed to heat, cold, deep pressure light pressure, vibration, and circumferential pressure, such as tight clothes). This is *not* the same as the physical therapy sensory rehabilitation most CRPS patients are used to, which focuses on continuing to expose the sensory nerves to a specific sensory stimulation, hoping to cause a "numbing down" effect after a while, almost like a callus. Instead, our system is based on the principle that the nervous system can self-heal if the injury is pointed out to the brain, and then the brain is gently assisted in fixing the glitch. Healing often occurs instantly, although reinjury may quickly happen in the beginning. The nervous system has to build up stamina and strength, at which point the corrections become permanent. In other words, this system toughens up your nervous system. It is like giving a soldier armor to wear, and it is very important if we send your body out into a world where it could potentially be reinjured.

Reinjury does not just mean *physical* injuries. Anything that puts stress on the nervous system may reinjure a fragile nervous system. Stress is defined as anything that changes the function of your body, even briefly. For example; eating a banana requires your body to make some changes and function in a certain way in order to digest it and eliminate its waste material. Therefore, even eating a banana is defined as a "stress." When the nervous system is newly recovered, it is very vulnerable to reinjury.

We encourage our patients to be very careful in the beginning phases of healing, even if they feel ready to take on the world. My golden rule is to do only 50 percent of what you feel you are (newly) capable of in the first five to six weeks of treatment. I have had some very enthusiastic patients over the years, and examples of reinjury include (but are not limited to) tilling a giant brand-new vegetable garden, riding a monstrous wooden roller-coaster, remodeling a library in two days, and babysitting twin babies overnight. I wish I could make this stuff up! Fortunately, some of our old patients who suffer from CRPS have really put their bodies to the test. We have had patients undergo surgery, involved in car accidents, and even fractured the original CRPS site. So far, none of these patients have reported reactivation or spreading of the CRPS symptoms.

FOURTH PUNCH: INCREASING CIRCULATION

The Vecttor was developed by Dr. Donald A. Rhodes, a podiatrist. While treating a postsurgical patient who developed CRPS, he discovered that at the time, there were no truly effective treatments available to treat this debilitating, painful condition. After many years of intense research and hard work, the Vecttor was cleared by the FDA as a treatment for chronic, intractable pain in November 2012. This therapy is unique as it constantly monitors the patient's temperature, and utilizes this feedback to deliver the best treatment.

Vecttor therapy is a form of electrostimulation utilizing the principles of acupuncture, refelexology, physiology, and cellular physiology designed to stimulate the nerves to produce certain vital neuropeptides essential for optional functioning of the body. Neuropeptides are small protein-like molecules used by the nerve cells in order to communicate with each other. They are involved in a wide range of nerve function, and are critical to the central nervous system's overall health. The Vecttor is *not* a TENS unit. The principal difference between a TENS unit and the Vecttor is that TENS uses a 10,000 Hertz frequency and Vecttor uses frequencies between 1 to 80 Hertz. This allows the Vecttor unit to stimulate special nerve cells called C-fiber nerve cells to release the nerve chemicals which decrease inflammation, normalize carbohydrate metabolism, and increase circulation at the cellular level throughout the body. This especially affects the autonomic nervous system.

OTHER THINGS

In addition to my "Four Punch" system, we do additional things to encourage healing. These include detoxification, treating the body to allergies to things like the patient's own blood, breaking up of scar tissue, and supplementation. As stated previously, our system works best when all components mentioned above are used together. There are no side effects to our treatment. Unfortunately, at this time, we are the only clinic in the United States to apply the "fourpunch" system. That means that you have to travel to Arkansas for ten weeks in order to get treated in our clinic.

As with anything, there are pros and cons to our system. While our success rate is high, we cannot help everybody. Our treatment is not covered by insurance, and you have to travel all the way to Arkansas to try it. The pros are obvious: no side effects, a high success rate, making the body healthier overall, and the ability to reasonably be able to predict if the treatment will work for you early on.

11

Give Your Body a Fighting Chance: Your Diet

Let your food be your medicine and your medicine your food.

—Hippocrates

One of the biggest tragedies of human civilization is the precedents of chemical therapy over nutrition. It's a substitution of chemical therapy over nature, of poisons over food, in which we are feeding people poisons trying to correct the reactions of starvation.

—Dr. Royal Lee

It is my belief that anyone who suffers from CRPS also suffers from global inflammation in the body. Inflammation increases your risk of getting cancer, autoimmune diseases, Alzheimer's disease, and many other diseases and conditions. It also ages you prematurely. If your body is already burdened on a daily basis by the horrific pain that is the benchmark of CRPS as well as the toxic environment created by daily medications, it does not need to be burdened by unhealthy foods as well. You would do your body a tremendous favor by decreasing the daily toxic burden it is under, by simply making changes to your diet. A lot of CRPS patients have told me that they simply do not have the energy left at the end of the day to afford spending that energy on trying to eat a healthy diet. The thing is you cannot afford *not* to.

That being said, I suggest that all changes are made very gradually. The reason for this is that if you dramatically change your diet overnight, you are at risk of undergoing a major detoxification reaction. What is a detoxification reaction exactly? As discussed in chapter 6, when you eat toxic and unhealthy food for a long time (not to mention also taking toxic medications), your liver and other detoxification organs and pathways (such as the kidneys, lymphatic system, and bowels) become overburdened. When this happens, the excess toxins are stored in your fat cells to get rid of later. When you start eating healthy, that day arrives, and your body starts processing massive amounts of backup toxins. However, this process is most often too much for the overburdened bodies of CRPS to handle and can not only flare your pain into monstrous proportions but also make you very sick. Start by changing one meal at a time. I suggest breakfast, first. After your body is used to this, you can start working on lunch and so on.

I believe that our body is a precious gift and that we have to be a good steward of it. We have an opportunity to either add to our health or detract from it every time we open our mouths to put food or liquid into them. After we swallow this food, it is now up to our body to either maximize the healing potential of the food we just ate or minimize the damage caused by it in the best way it can, until it gets too tired to do so. If you suffer from CRPS, you need the support that good nutritious food can give you even more than the average person and can afford damage from bad food even less.

The problem is if you are like most people, you are probably as confused as a chameleon in a bag of Skittles about what exactly you should or should not eat. As you have so much on your plate, it is my sincere belief that a healthy diet should follow sound principles and be kept simple. Healthy eating should be so simple that you can follow it most days of the rest of your life. Give a man a fish, and you feed him for a day; teach a man to fish, and you feed him for a lifetime.

With that in mind, we will explain some broad principles, followed by some daily food suggestions and suggestions of things to avoid, such as a toxic friend.

Keep it simple, stupid.

—Kelly Johnson

WHAT IS YOUR PH? ACID VERSUS ALKALINE

If you ever took even the most basic chemistry class, you probably know that any liquid has either an alkaline or an acid pH. Our bodies were designed to be alkaline by nature (at a tightly controlled pH of 7.4) and acidic by function—meaning that the waste products our cells produce when they work are usually acidic. Your alkalinity is determined not only by your diet but also by the toxins you are exposed to, the air that you breathe, the liquids you drink, how much you exercise, and even your thoughts.

The stability of your blood pH is protected from swings, since even a tiny swing in pH may kill you. In fact, this is a major argument by those who oppose the acid/alkaline principle. According to them, your blood is protected from swings in pH and therefore should not be affected by an acidic diet. While that is true, when it comes to your urine (and the rest of your body), it is a different story. When your diet is very acidic, your urine chemistry is altered in profound ways, possibly resulting in kidney stones, which you may have heard aren't much fun.

When your diet is mostly acidic, it takes a big toll on your body. It will cause cellular inflammation (the last thing you need) and aging, and besides the aforementioned kidney stones, it may also cause gallstones and osteoporosis, the latter taking place because your body will basically "dissolve" bones in order to buffer the acid. Think of your bones as a bank. When your diet is too acidic, your body has to "borrow" calcium from your bones in order to buffer it, with every intention of "paying back" this loan once you clean up your act. The problem is most people never do.

An acidic diet will also decrease the body's ability to repair damaged cells as well as its ability to absorb minerals and other nutrients. This results in a decrease in the energy production of the cells, lowering their ability to detoxify heavy metals and other toxins. This may cause cancer cells to thrive and make the body more vulnerable to fatigue, general wear and tear, and illness.

On the other hand, your health will greatly improve if your diet is more alkaline. Your skin will look younger (remember, osteoporosis has been tied to the appearance of wrinkles), your bones will be stronger, and you will be less likely to be overweight.

It is fairly simple to test your saliva and urine pH at home armed with some pH paper, and I recommend that every person with CRPS do it. For a more detailed guide to this testing, you may go here: http://www.energiseforlife.com/wordpress/2006/04/12/alkaline-test-how-to-test-your-ph-levels-saliva-urine/. For a complete list of acid/alkaline foods, you can easily turn to Google.

For the most part, vegetables and fruits (and most nuts and seeds) are alkaline, and animal products, such as meat and cheese, refined carbs, junk food, sugar, and pastas are acidic foods. As a general rule, if you are sick, you should aim for an 80/20 balance, where 80 percent of the food you eat has an alkaline pH or effect on the body (for instance, even though a lemon is acidic, it will have an alkalizing *effect* on your body). Please be advised that your body might be so excited because of this change that it may actually start "spring cleaning" and detoxifying old piled-up toxins.

As discussed earlier in this chapter, this may not feel too pleasant and can often not be tolerated by those who suffer from CRPS. If this happens—in the form of diarrhea, headaches, or a general unpleasant feeling—back off from the alkaline food, and go about it more slowly. You will have to find your own pace. In order to *maintain* health, a 70/30 (70 percent alkaline foods, 30 percent acid foods) daily balance is recommended. A great supplement to alkalize your body on a daily basis is green barley powder.

Remember, it's OK to mess up some of the time, as long as you eat good, mostly alkaline food most of the time. No one is taking away your ice cream forever!

IT'S ALL ABOUT OMEGA-3/OMEGA-6S

There are two types of fats essential to your body, omega-3 and omega-6. However, the typical modern human being consumes far too many omega-6 fats in his or her diet while consuming very low levels of omega-3. The primary sources of omega-6 are soy, corn, grape seed, canola, safflower, and sunflower oils. These oils are used in tons of mass-produced food and fast food and are overabundant in the typical diet, which explains our excess omega-6 levels. Avoid or limit these oils. Omega-3, meanwhile, is typically found in flaxseed, virgin coconut, krill, and fish oils.

By far, the best type of omega-3 fats are those found in that last category—fish. That's because the omega-3 in fish is high in two fatty acids crucial to human health, DHA and EPA. These two fatty acids are pivotal in preventing heart disease, cancer, and many other diseases. Unfortunately, the ocean has become a more contaminated environment, and care must be taken to avoid the intake of heavy metals together with your fish oil. Do not buy cheap fish-oil supplements at large stores. For recommended brands, please go to "Fish Oil" in chapter 12.

Remember, the ideal ratio of omega-6 to omega-3 fats is 1:1, a ratio maintained by our ancestors for millions of years. Today, though, according to Dr. Mercola and other sources, our ratio of omega-6 to omega-3 averages anywhere from 20:1 to 50:1! This imbalance may contribute to autoimmune conditions, cancer, pain, Alzheimer's disease, and cellular inflammation (of particular concern for those who suffer from CRPS), to name a few. In your case, it is crucial that you work toward a healthier omega-3/omega-6 balance, since this is one of the main tools in fighting inflammation.

YOUR CELLS ON FIRE: THE ROLE OF CELLULAR INFLAMMATION

Let's do a quick recap on inflammation. Inflammation is the normal expected immune response of tissues due to any injury. Signs of acute inflammation include heat, pain, swelling, and redness at the site of the injury. Your body may also become stiff in one area (e.g., a sprained ankle joint), thereby protecting the joint from excessive movements while it is healing (remember how smart your body is?). This type of acute inflammation is normally a localized, protective, logical response following infection or trauma.

However, if the agent causing the inflammation persists for a prolonged period of time, the inflammation becomes chronic, as in the case of CRPS. People who suffer from autoimmune conditions and allergies are particularly vulnerable to exaggerated inflammatory responses.

Inflammation may be fought through a healthy diet relatively low in protein, including good quality protein, healthy oils and fats, lots of fruits and vegetables, plenty of omega-3s (restoring the balance in the central nervous system), and supplementation. It is also *crucial* to rebuild the gut in order to decrease cellular inflammation (addressed later in this book).

Stay in the range of 40 g (for women) to 55 g (for men) of animal protein a day (unless you are an Olympic athlete).

(These numbers were obtained by the CDC [Centers for Disease Control]. Children's required protein intake may fall anywhere between 13 and 40 grams depending on their age). Note that pregnant women also require higher daily intakes of protein.

The more protein you eat, the more calcium you lose in your urine. Also, remember that a major goal for those who suffer from CRPS is to cut down on cellular inflammation (see above). Excess protein will cause cellular inflammation.

Good quality protein is far more important than quantity. We recommend healthy whey in smoothies as a great source of protein (go to mercola.com for whey recommendations) or a product called "Dream Protein," available on Amazon.com.

Putting Out the Fire

You are what you eat, so don't be fast, easy, cheap, or fake.

—U<small>NKNOWN</small>

ANIMALS ARE WHAT THEY EAT: TRY TO KEEP YOUR ANIMAL PRODUCTS NATURAL

Study after study has shown that the omega-3/omega-6 balances in grain-fed animals, such as bison, chicken, and beef, are not healthy. When you eat beef, make sure that it is grass-fed beef. The longer cattle eat grain, the greater the fatty-acid imbalance (omega-3/omega-6) in their meat. After even two hundred days (standard in the United States), it has been shown that omega-6/omega-3 ratios may exceed 20 to 1. Venison is generally better for you than beef, unless the deer was exposed to soy.

Also, make sure that when you eat eggs or chicken or turkey, you only consume the eggs or meat of chicken and turkey that eat vegetables high in omega-3 fats, along with insects and grass, supplemented with fruit and very small amounts of corn. According to Dr. Mercola, range-fed eggs have an omega-6 /omega-3 ratio of 1.5 to 1, whereas the egg you typically buy at a supermarket has a ratio of 20 to 1. Please avoid "omega-3 enriched" eggs. While this sounds like a good idea in theory, these chickens are usually not fed in a healthy way.

Farm-raised fish, such as tilapia and catfish, have been found to be especially detrimental to your health, based on at least one study of its effect on your omega-3/omega-6 ratio.[57] Some people even call tilapia the "bacon of the ocean" because of this. Make sure that, as a rule, the fish you eat is not farm-raised, as the emphasis in the industry is to get these fish produced in mass quantities and to breed them to be as large as possible.

WATCH THOSE CARBS

Few other areas in nutrition have been debated as hotly and passionately as carbohydrates. At least one major Japanese study found that the intelligence and actual anatomy of the brains of schoolchildren were altered based on the amount and type of carbs they consumed in the morning for breakfast.[58] Another study found a direct link between refined carbs and an increased risk of stroke in women.[59]

How healthy or unhealthy a specific carb usually depends upon its glycemic index (GI) or how fast that specific carb raises your blood sugar after eating it relative to pure glucose (which has a GI of one hundred). Generally, the higher the GI, the worse the food is for you, the faster it raises your insulin, and the more inflammation it causes. While I am not a big believer in completely cutting out an entire food group, I do believe that it will benefit CRPS patients especially to limit their carbohydrate consumption to about two servings of healthy carbohydrates a day.

Carbs are actually the one food group not essential for survival. However, as we said before, we prefer moderation instead of elimination. Your body much prefers getting its carbs from fruits and vegetables, as they have a low GI and release blood sugar slowly. Try to limit your intake of healthy grains (let's call them moderate carbs) to no more than 20 percent of your daily diet. These include all those carbs that you were probably taught were essential for health, including brown and white rice, barley, potatoes, corn, millet, nuts, and whole-grain bread.

Try to eliminate unhealthy carbs (bad carbs) as much as you can, except as a special treat every now and then. Pretend that bad carps are like toxic exes. Contact should be limited. I am not telling you to bake a hemp cake decorated with nuts for your birthday, but just to be good most of the time. Unhealthy carbs include white bread, bagels, pretzels, and anything looking irresistible at your local bakery (doughnuts, cream puffs, and croissants, for instance) as well as processed cakes and treats like Twinkies (yes, they are coming back) and so on. This group also includes sugar, high-fructose corn syrup, and fructose. Please use honey or stevia (a natural sweetener) instead.

As an added bonus, cutting down on your carbs will positively affect your health as well as your weight. Cutting down on carbs seems to be especially beneficial for those who suffer from neuropathic pain, as discussed below.

AVOID CARBS AND BRING ON THE FAT: KETOGENIC DIET

At least one major study has shown that chronic pain and inflammation responds extremely well to a ketogenic diet (Ketogenic diets and pain, Journal of child neurology, 2013). What is a ketogenic diet? Basically, the biggest factor in whether a diet is ketogenic or not is how low the carbohydrate intake is. Generally, those who suffer from severe chronic neurologic pain (such as CRPS) want to eat fewer than 50mg of carbs/day. Ketosis means that your body is in a state where it doesn't have enough glucose to use as energy, and metabolizes fat instead. During this process, special molecules called ketones are generated. Therefor, the basis of this diet is to eat LOTS of healthy fats and oils (grass-fed butter, olive oil, coconut oil, animal fats, avocado, etc.) as well as vegetables (raw is best) and protein in moderation.

In addition to pain, there is strong evidence that obesity, type 2 diabetes, epilepsy, and heart problems all majorly benefit from a ketogenic diet. There is emerging evidence that many neurological diseases, such as brain trauma and Alzheimer's disease, also respond well to it.

Switching to a ketogenic diet may be difficult at first, as you will go through a one to two-week withdrawal process where you miss your carbs like a beloved ex. After this initial period, your body does adjust, however. For more info on ketogenic diets, you may go to realmealrevolution.com

BOTTOMS UP

We have all heard that we need eight eight-ounce glasses of water every day. However, this information is outdated. The Institute of Medicine set its general guidelines for women to consume a total of ninety-one ounces (about two point seven liters) per day. For men, it's about one hundred and twenty-five ounces a day (or three point seven liters). Keep in mind that those numbers include water from all the food and beverages you consume combined. Depending on your diet, about 25 percent of the water you consume comes from your food. The simplest way to tell whether you drink enough water is to look at your urine. It should be light yellow (unless you take vitamins or supplements affecting the color). It should also not have a strong odor.

Hate drinking water? You are not alone. We can actually dampen our desire for water (thirsting mechanism) over time if our bodies get accustomed to constant dehydration. Age can also have this affect. Don't be fooled, however. Every cell in your body needs water.

When it comes to what kind of water to drink, always ask yourself, "What would nature do?" We do not recommend that you drink water straight out of a faucet due to additives and toxicity issues. Ionized water is alkalized by electricity splitting the water molecules, without added minerals. In nature, water flows over rocks and through soil, collecting naturally alkalizing minerals, such as calcium and magnesium. If you drink this type of water, be sure to add trace minerals or lemon juice to your water (more about that in a bit). Also, never drink water that is too alkaline (pH above eight), as your body will counter this by acidifying itself.

Avoid bottled water in plastic bottles unless the bottle is BPA free, as BPA (a harmful chemical found in plastics) often leaches into the water, especially if heated up (never leave bottled water in a hot car). Distilled and reverse osmosis water is "dead" water that will leach minerals from your body. Always add the juice of half a lemon to filtered water, as this will add minerals back into the water and is also naturally alkalizing. (Do rinse your mouth out after with plain water in order to protect your teeth). You may also add trace minerals in liquid form.

IT TAKES MORE THAN ONE APPLE A DAY

Unless you have been living under a rock, you have probably heard that fruits and veggies are good for you. As a general rule, you should try to eat five to seven cups of fruits and vegetables a day. Vegetables and fruits will lower your risk of heart disease, stroke, osteoporosis, certain kinds of cancers, kidney and gallstones, and oxidative stress, and they increase your mental clarity.[60,61] They also contain enzymes that assist digestion and are full of antioxidants and phytochemicals that help to boost your immune system.

Eating your fruits and veggies has also been shown to be very beneficial to those who suffer from chronic conditions (of particular interest to you). As a general rule, vegetables rebuild your cells, and fruits clean (detoxify) them. One study, reviewing two hundred other studies studying the relationship between fruits and vegetables and cancer, found overwhelming evidence that "persons with low fruit and vegetable intake (at least the lower one-fourth of the population) experience about twice the risk of cancer compared with those with high intake, even after control for potentially confounding factors."[62]

Because most people with chronic diseases are also somewhat insulin resistant, it is best to keep your fruit/vegetable ratio at 30 percent fruit to 70 percent vegetables. A few additional things to remember: raw is always best (keeping the enzymes, nutrients, and alkalinity intact), and, for my readers from the South, where nothing is above frying, deep-frying it pretty much turns any vegetable into the equivalent of a doughnut. Also, potatoes aren't vegetables, and while buying all organic is certainly too expensive for most of us, I really do suggest that you avoid "dirty" fruits and vegetables, since eating them does more harm than good, unless you buy them organic. On the other hand, you may buy "clean" produce anywhere.

- **Dirty fruits**
  Peaches, cherries, apples, nectarines, strawberries, grapes (imported), and pears
- **Clean fruits**
  Cantaloupes, grapefruit, kiwifruit, mangoes, papayas, and pineapples
- **Dirty vegetables**
  Bell peppers, celery, kale, lettuce, carrots, cherry tomatoes, cucumbers, hot peppers, potatoes (technically a starch), spinach, collard greens, and summer squash
- **Clean vegetables**
  Avocadoes, asparagus, cabbage, sweet peas, sweet corn, eggplant, mushrooms, onions, and sweet potatoes

Everything not on these lists and not certified organic should be treated with suspicion and peeled or washed when possible. To make your own vegetable wash, combine equal amounts of white vinegar and clean water. Mix and spray onto hard-skinned produce, or soak soft-skinned produce for two minutes in the solution in a bowl. Rinse under a faucet.

> **Tip: Get into a habit of making one or two smoothies every day. This way it is easier to consume larger amounts of produce in its raw form and to get the needed servings every day. For breakfast, I use a Vitamix® blender (worth its weight in gold, although any good blender will work) and add one or two fruits, such as orange, lemon, lime, blueberries, pineapple, and apple, four or five vegetables, such as kale, spinach, beets, carrots, and even radishes with water, whey powder (grass-fed), coconut oil, flaxseed oil, fish oil (undetected by taste if of superior quality), cinnamon, and ginger root. Experiment with the tastes you like, and start with more fruits to acclimate to the taste.**

FATS DON'T MAKE YOU FAT.

Let me repeat that. *Fats don't make you fat.*

One of the worse rumors that ever got started regarding food is that fat is bad for you and leads to heart attacks and strokes and will cause you to have a body that is less than svelte. Healthy fats are crucial for those who suffer from inflammation and chronic pain (see Avoid carbs and bring on the fat: Ketogenic diet, above)

Eating a low-fat diet was believed to be the holy grail of healthful eating and low cholesterol for decades. Seeing a fantastic marketing opportunity, and also giving the public what it wanted, food companies reinvented and reengineered thousands of foods to be lower in fat or fat free, often increasing the salt, sugar, or chemicals in these foods to make up for lost flavor.

Fats provide essential fatty acids, which are not made by the body and must be obtained from food. The essential fatty acids (linoleic and linolenic acid) are necessary for many biological processes in the body, such as vitamin and mineral absorption (why it is good to take vitamin D together with healthy fat or oil), revving up your metabolism (that's right, weight loss!), brain function, fighting cellular inflammation, heart health, and many more.[63]

When it comes to being bad for you or fattening, it is not the amount of fats that count but the quality and types. In addition to the 1:1 omega-3/omega-6 balance we already discussed, you also need some other fats. Let's look at an overview of those to eat and those to avoid and the categories these fats are divided into.

SATURATED FATS

Some are good, and some are bad, such as butter (limit), ice cream (limit), cream (limit), fatty meats (fine if grass-fed), avocado (good for you), nuts (good for you, with the exception of peanut butter), and coconut (it is good for you *if* of good quality and virgin and great for cooking, as it is not very much damaged by heat; make sure that it smells like coconuts). If you have heard that coconut oil is bad for you, that information is outdated and incorrect, as most old studies on coconut oil used hydrogenated or partially hydrogenated coconut oil.

UNSATURATED FATS

Unsaturated fats are divided into monounsaturated fats (olive and canola oils) and polyunsaturated fats (sunflower, fish, safflower, corn, and soybean oils). Of the above list, we prefer using olive oil (best if not heated above 250°F/121°C) and fish oil.

HYDROGENATED AND PARTIALLY HYDROGENATED FATS

Hydrogenation is the chemical process by which liquid saturated oils are turned into solid fat. In other words, these are hardened or partially hardened oils (such as hard butter). Foods containing hydrogenated oils should be avoided because they contain high levels of trans-fatty acids, which are linked to heart disease, increased "bad" cholesterol (LDL), and decreased "good" cholesterol (HDL).

TRANS-FATTY ACIDS

These fats form when hydrogen atoms are added to an unsaturated fat, such as vegetable oil (hydrogenation), and can raise LDL ("bad" cholesterol) and lower HDL levels ("good cholesterol"). Trans-fatty acids are found in fried foods, commercial baked goods (doughnuts, cookies, crackers, chips), processed foods, and margarines.

You get the general idea. Higher omega-3s and lower omega-6s are good, some saturated fats are good and even necessary (contrary to long-held popular belief), most unsaturated fats are good (but shouldn't be heated as a general rule), and hydrogenated, partially hydrogenated, and trans fats should be avoided as diligently as swimsuit models avoid cream puffs.

ALLERGIES AND OTHER IRRITATING FOODS

People who suffer from CRPS almost always suffer from food allergies, resulting from a "confused" immune system and a digestive system not working properly, leaking large particles into the bloodstream, where they are attacked by the immune system as foreign particles. While we are huge proponents of first restoring proper nervous-system communication and then rebuilding the digestive systems of those who suffer from CRPS, it is crucial to stop pouring irritating foods into that system. This is especially true because foods that cause an allergic reaction in those who suffer from CRPS will also increase inflammation.

If there is a specific food that you crave, like sugar, there is a good chance that you are allergic to that food. Isn't that a strange oxymoron? It is theorized that the reason this happens is that when a food allergy causes chemical and physical stress inside your body, your body produces endorphins, which comfort you and make you feel good, thus making you crave more for it. One of my vices is Starbucks coffee. I find myself especially craving for it when my energy is low or I am emotionally in a bad spot, just as a treat or a pick-me-up.

Allergies to food will make the whole repair process rather ineffective, like a dog chasing its own tail. Also, it will increase cellular inflammation and therefore pain. First, get a proper blood test to determine which foods you are allergic to. I suggest that you get tested for food-specific reactions to three different antibodies: IgG, IgE, and IgA, which typically result from noticeable reactions to specific foods.

One of the ways your immune system defends against invaders, such as viruses, bacteria, or a foreign particle, is by producing cells called antibodies, also called immunoglobulins. There are five major immunoglobulins: IgA, IgD, IgE, IgG, and IgM.

Only IgE reactions are considered true food *allergies* and will require a blood draw. IgE reactions typically occur within minutes of exposure to or ingestion of a specific food. Common IgE reactions include trouble breathing, wheezing, flushing, a feeling of getting hot, hives, itchy watery eyes, swelling, and anxiety. Testing for IgE food allergies requires a blood draw.

Food sensitivity is a term that usually refers to delayed immune reactions to foods, or nonimmune reactions to food. The symptoms of food sensitivities and allergies are quite different. While a food allergy normally causes an immediate reaction, the symptoms of food sensitivities may not be as obvious as those of food allergies. The reasons for this are that often food sensitivities are delayed and the reactions are not as clearly identifiable.

The following are just a few examples of symptoms of food sensitivities: fatigue, lethargy, anger, exhaustion (especially after eating), headaches, migraines, mood swings, depression, restlessness, water retention, joint pain, gas, bloating, constipation, diarrhea, and indigestion. IgG and IgA react to foods and can be detected from a dry strip sample of blood.

Eight foods cause 90 percent of all allergies in the United States. These are peanuts, tree nuts (such as walnuts), milk, eggs, wheat, soy, fish, and shellfish.

In addition, people who suffer from chronic pain have been shown to be sensitive to nightshade vegetables. Nightshade fruits and vegetables are said to grow "in the shade of the night" (rather creepy, if you ask me) and contain chemicals such as alkaloids that can increase arthritic pain and symptoms. The most common nightshades are potatoes, tomatoes, peppers (sweet and hot), eggplant, tomatillos, pimentos (usually used to stuff olives), cherries, paprika, and cayenne.

Golden rule: Try to eat well 80 percent of the time, and allow yourself to mess up 20 percent of the time. Striving for excellence is more sustainable than striving for perfection.

THE EXCEPTION TO THE 80/20 RULE: THE NO-NO LIST

Trust me, the following foods are not worth the harm they cause you. They are toxic, nasty, cancer-causing, pain-elevating, hormone-disrupting, and generally wreak havoc upon your body. To make this list, these chemicals and additives had to be particularly offensive to your health and well-being.

The culprits are as follows:

- Artificial sweeteners (as discussed in chapter 4) such as aspartame (NutraSweet, Equal), saccharin (Sweet'N' Low, SugarTwin), and sucralose (Splenda)
- Diet sodas and chewing gum containing these sweeteners
- High-fructose corn syrup
- Artificial coloring agents (usually a color followed by a number, such as FD&C Blue No. 1) that have been shown by at least one study to interfere with your body's energy (ATP) production,[64] already a problem area in those with CRPS
- Monosodium glutamate (MSG)
- Major hormone-disrupting butylatedhydroxyanisole (BHA) and butylatedhydroxytoluene (BHT)

- Sodium nitrite and sodium nitrate (potentially linked to diabetes and colon cancer)
- Potassium bromate (potentially carcinogenic and illegal in Canada, Europe, China, and Brazil)
- Recombinant bovine growth hormone (rBGH)
- Sodium benzoate and potassium benzoate (benzene is a known carcinogen that is also linked with serious thyroid damage, especially if, e.g., soda bottles in plastic containing benzene are exposed to heat in transport)

So remember, don't try to be perfect, be excellent. Stop eating mindlessly and conveniently. Educate yourself so that you can learn how to make healthy choices on your own, and you can be like a strong oak tree, not swayed this way or that by the media every time a new wind of change or nutritional fad blows through. You must arm yourself with basic nutritional knowledge and daily habits that will withstand the test of time and that will allow you to feed and honor your body with the best kind of medicine there is: healthy, nutritious food.

12

The Supplement Maze: Where to Begin?

The doctor of the future will give no medicine but will interest the patient in the care of the human frame, in diet, and in the cause and prevention of disease.

—THOMAS EDISON

Supplement: *something that is added to something else in order to make it complete.*

—MERRIAM-WEBSTER

Few things are as confusing as knowing which supplements to take every day. If you are like most CRPS patients, there is a good chance that you have probably already spent a fortune on supplements and natural potions. Most well-meaning people, if they know that you are not well, will bring the newest gimmicky supplement to your attention. Ditto if you sell the special newest multimarketing you-can-only-pick-these-in-the-Andes-after-four-days-on-the-back-of-a-donkey mountain berry juice. People who don't feel well are easy targets. Sure, the fact that you have only heard about this on late-night infomercials made you suspicious, but you were hurting and desperate, and it wouldn't hurt to try, right?

The problem is it hurts your pocket, and sometimes all you are doing is adding expensive supplements to your urine. They may pass right through you unabsorbed, they may not benefit you, and they may even harm you. This is especially the case if you suffer from cellular inflammation, as this makes the cell membrane hard and impermeable. What this means is that a lot of the (often expensive) supplements you take never even make it into your cells. It's as if your cells are surrounded by water, yet dying of thirst.

Allopathic doctors are generally not very well versed when it comes to vitamins, minerals, or supplements. Up until very recently, recommending vitamins was still frowned upon by the AMA as nonscientific, unconventional, or a form of quackery. Medical schools still do not teach much about diet or supplementation. This is especially true in the world that CRPS patients move in. The focus is not on whole body health but on effective pain management at any cost, often leaving your detoxification organs, like the liver, to suffer in the wake of this approach. Your body is beat up not only by CRPS but also by its management.

> *In medical school I had not received any significant instruction on the subject. I was not alone. Only approximately 6 percent of the graduating physicians in the United States have any training in nutrition. Medical students may take elective courses on the topic, but few actually do...the education of most physicians is disease-oriented with a heavy emphasis on pharmaceuticals—we learn about drugs and why and when to use them.*
>
> —RAY D. STRAND, MD, THE AUTHOR OF DEATH BY PRESCRIPTION

Scientific studies on supplements and vitamins are hard to find, and you won't find many medical journals publishing papers about natural vitamins and supplements. The reason for this is that a decent study is very, very expensive and some entity, corporation, or interest group usually has to have a financial or other incentive to pay for these studies. Vitamins are not patentable, so drug companies can't just sell a vitamin the way it appears in nature. In order to be patented so that they won't lose all the millions of dollars they have invested in it, it has to be altered somehow or made unique.

I have noticed a trend on the Internet: if someone speaks out about something that works, the collective response from other people suffering from the same condition is "show us the research." Even natural or alternative health-care providers may greatly disagree when it comes to what is or isn't needed or what is or isn't good. When I set out on my quest to learn how to help people who suffer from chronic pain, I was especially daunted by supplementation. Just when you think you are comfortable in this field, a new study comes out, contradicting something you were certain before was right.

When I set out to learn how to add nutrition and supplements to my treatment regimen, I didn't have time to reinvent the wheel. I had to find the best and learn from them. When I chose my teachers, I looked at some of the same criteria that I think patients should examine when picking a doctor. How healthy do they appear themselves? Smart doctors follow their own advice. If someone's regime works, it should show in their figure, their skin, and their general vitality. Also, what are their verifiable patient outcomes? Do their patients actually respond to their care?

Based on all the collective knowledge I have gathered over the years from these teachers and nutritional industry experts, I have narrowed my list of vitamins down to the most beneficial and essential. Below is a list of some of the supplements and vitamins that I believe may be helpful to those who suffer from CRPS. Please note that this is not a complete list, as such a list would need a book of its own. Also, this is meant as a guide only and not meant to replace the advice of your doctor.

Lastly, it is not my belief that supplements or vitamins can "cure" CRPS. Remember, I don't even like to use the word "cure." However, your poor body suffers every day from indescribable levels of pain, and supplements can *help*. Pain fatigues your every cell and places an undue burden on the body. Your body will find it very difficult to fight CRPS in this state. If there is any chance of you beating this monster, your body will need all the support you can give it. One excellent way to provide this support is through taking great nutrition as well as taking the correct vitamins and supplements. In addition, you don't want to add other conditions on top of the CRPS.

It is important that you clear every supplement you take with your doctor, as it may negatively interact with medications that you are taking. If you can find a doctor knowledgeable in applied kinesiology (or muscle testing), you can make sure that you only take the supplements that will specifically be beneficial to you. Many alternative health-care providers have been trained in this skill.

Occasionally, you will notice that I recommend a *specific* vitamin or supplement. When I do so, it is merely because I am familiar and satisfied with that supplement's performance. Rest assured that I am receiving absolutely no financial reward for promoting specific supplements.

All diseases or conditions, from cancer to CRPS, have the following in common: a body with an acidic pH; oxidation of the body; inflammation of the body; and a body that is tired, overloaded, and breaking down. Since we are surrounded by toxins and often overloading out body with chemicals, it is most important that you arm your body on a daily basis, optimizing it and making it strong in order to handle any stress thrown at it, be it physical, chemical, or emotional.

WHOLE-FOOD MULTIVITAMIN

It is my opinion that you should take more than the recommended dose (with the exception of iron and a few fat-soluble vitamins listed below), preferably a few in the morning and a

> *few with lunch or dinner. Do not exceed the recommended dose of iron for the day, which is 10 mg for males and 10–15 mg for females. Also, watch out for exceeding the maximum daily recommended intake for vitamin A (10,000 IU) and vitamin E (1,500 IU).*

Even if you are a healthy eater, it is very difficult to get all the vitamins your body needs today just from your food and beverages. When it comes to a multivitamin, you must choose quality and be prepared to pay a bit more in order to obtain that quality. If you buy your vitamins in a big chain supermarket or pharmacy, chances are that they won't be of superior quality. The companies that manufacture discount vitamins usually use cheap synthetic isolates (incomplete vitamins) combined with chemicals. Your body only absorbs parts of these vitamins, and what is absorbed can't really be used.

Any multivitamin that promises that one a day will be enough is usually a giant waste of money. Even though technology is amazing today, it is still impossible to compress all the vitamins and minerals your body needs into one tiny pill.

> *Please make sure that any multivitamin you take contains fewer than 100 mcg (i.e., micrograms, not macro!) of copper. Why is this so crucial? Copper has been linked to dementia. A six-year study of more than three thousand seven hundred people sixty-five or older showed that those who consumed at least 1.6 milligrams of copper a day added almost twenty years to their ages in terms of mental decline.*[65]

I recommend Dr. Mercola's Multivitamin Plus® (www.mercola.com). He also gives a children's vitamin, but my favorite multivitamin for children is by Natural Vitality: Kid's Natural Calm Multi Liquid® (www.naturalvitality.com, or call 866-416-9216).

VITAMIN D3

Most people are Vitamin D3 deficient, especially in the winter months. According to Dr. Mercola, It's important to regularly measure your vitamin D levels to make sure you're maintaining therapeutic levels of 50–70 ng/mL year-round. There are two vitamin D tests: 1,25(OH)D and 25(OH)D. The correct test is 25(OH)D, also called 25-hydroxyvitamin D. This is the better marker of overall D status, and is most strongly associated with overall health. If you live in the United States, Dr. Mercola recommends that you use either tests done by Lab Corp or the blood-spot test that grassrootshealth.net uses.

In the summer, you may need 2,000–5,000 IU, or you may need 5,000–8,000 IU if you do not spend much time in the sun. In the winter, you may need up to 10,000 IU. If you are depleted, you may need anywhere from 10,000 to 20,000 IU for six months to catch up. You will find that this is well above commonly recommended daily vitamin D3 intake. If you are taking these high quantities of vitamin D3, it is vital that you also take vitamin K2. Usually, studies that dispute higher recommended daily intake of vitamin D3 ignore the role of vitamin K2, greatly affecting the outcome of those studies and essentially invalidating them. More on this little-known vitamin will follow shortly.

When your body is exposed to UVB radiation from the sun, it forms vitamin D3, an oil-soluble steroid hormone. However, in today's world, where we do not spend much time outside and wear sunblock when we do go outside and where winter months can rob us from sunshine, most people are vitamin D3 deficient. Vitamin D3 is also found in animal organs and fat, cod-liver oil, fish, soymilk, and eggs. It is equivalent to the vitamin D3 your body makes when it's exposed to sunshine. You should stay away from the synthetic D2, as it has been shown to be highly toxic at the higher dosages.

Vitamin D3 is absolutely critical for overall good health and disease prevention. It is a major player in cancer prevention. It also positively affects the immune system, autoimmune conditions, insulin, bone density, blood pressure, genetic material, and almost all your organs. Actually, it would probably be easier to list the things vitamin D3 doesn't do than its benefits, since they are so numerous and widespread. A groundbreaking report suggests that taking vitamin D3 supplements may even reduce overall mortality rates: an in-depth analysis of multiple studies found that taking even modest levels of vitamin D supplements was associated with a statistically significant 7 percent reduction in mortality from any cause.[66] Simply put, vitamin D3 will apparently help you live longer. That is enough motivation to take it for me!

VITAMIN K2 (YOUR CALCIUM TAXI)

Adults typically need about 800–1,000 micrograms of this vitamin per day. Most people are vitamin K2 deficient.

Vitamin K is actually a group of three fat-soluble vitamins. The two main ones are K1 and K2; the third is K3. Chances are you have only heard of vitamin K1, which is found in green leafy vegetables, such as kale, broccoli, and spinach, and is very easy to get through your diet. K2 is harder to get and is found in butter, fermented foods, such as sauerkraut, and animal products, such as goose liver, ground beef, and chicken. (This lack of distinction has created a lot of confusion, and it's one of the reasons why vitamin K2 has been neglected for so long.) Vitamin K2 is also produced by bacteria in the colon that convert vitamin K1 into vitamin K2.

K2 prevents cancer (such as liver, prostate, and non-Hodgkin's lymphoma), helps to keep your arteries unblocked, and also works like a taxi for calcium, since it helps to move the calcium where your body needs it most, like your bones and your teeth. Actually, because of that function, you could say that this little-known vitamin is the missing link in fighting osteoporosis. One recent study found that vitamin K2 reduces fractures due to osteoporosis up to a whopping 87 percent.[67]

Because of this, it is crucial that if you are supplementing with vitamin D3 or getting lots of sunshine, you also take vitamin K2. Failure to do so may lead to calcification (e.g., of your arteries) due to inappropriate calcium deposits.

GLUTATHIONE

The amount of glutathione you should take depends upon the form in which you take it. Please follow the manufacturer's recommendation unless otherwise instructed by your doctor.

If supplements are boxers, think of glutathione as Rocky Balboa. Glutathione is a tripeptide (a substance that forms when three amino acids link together in a specific order). It is the most powerful antioxidant in your body's arsenal against cancer and toxicity. Because CRPS patients are often highly toxic and many cannot detoxify properly due to the MTHFR gene mutation, this supplement is especially crucial for these patients.

Glutathione is a unique antioxidant, since it works *within* the cell rather than from the outside. It maximizes all your other antioxidants, such as vitamin C. As you may be aware, antioxidants eliminate toxins and free radicals from your body. They are also one of your main defense systems against cancer. Glutathione protects the mitochondria in cells against oxidation.

Mitochondria: Mitochondria is the cell's powerhouse, producing energy used to fuel the functions of a cell.

Oxidation: Oxidation is the collective burden placed on cells by the constant production of free radicals in the normal course of metabolism plus whatever other toxins you are exposing your body to on a daily basis.

Glutathione strengthens your immune system, protects you from aging, and plays a major role in DNA repair. Glutathione deficiency has been linked to cancer, Alzheimer's, and many other conditions.

Unfortunately, it is very difficult for your body to absorb glutathione from your digestive system into your blood. For this reason, please beware of buying oral glutathione supplements, as they are most likely a waste of your money. Glutathione IVs are effective but not practical for everyone, although certainly worth it. Glutathione suppositories are the next best thing (although granted, nobody's favorite route of delivery). Only about 20 percent of it is absorbed through the skin. According to Dr. Mercola, the overall top food for maximizing your glutathione is high-quality *whey protein.* It must be cold-pressed whey protein derived from grass-fed cows, and free of hormones, chemicals, and sugar. Quality whey provides all the key amino acids for glutathione production (cysteine, glycine, and glutamate) and contains a unique cysteine residue (glutamylcysteine) that is highly bioactive in its affinity for converting to glutathione." We recommend that you add whey to smoothies.

Another way you can boost glutathione is by taking the building blocks that make glutathione, thereby boosting your glutathione production. These include the following.

N-ACETYL CYSTEINE

Take 600 mg tablets or capsules, twice daily. If you drink whey, try to take the NAC with your whey.

NAC is a slightly modified version of the sulfur-containing amino acid cysteine. It is a powerful free-radical scavenger, and therefore it decreases cellular inflammation. When taken internally, NAC replenishes intracellular levels of the natural antioxidant glutathione, helping to restore cells' ability to fight damage from free radicals. NAC boosts the immune system, protects against the flu, fights oxidation, decreases inflammation, fights the bad bacteria *Helicobacter pylori*, which cause stomach ulcers, and is responsible for a host of other benefits. It has been shown by at least one study to be helpful for CRPS.[68]

Take 600 mg tablets or capsules, twice daily.

ALPHA LIPOIC ACID

Alpha lipoic acid is required about 1,200 mg a day.

It is a fatty acid and a very powerful antioxidant. It destroys free radicals like nobody's business, can function in fat as well as water, and is the only known antioxidant that can get into the brain past the blood-brain barrier. Alpha lipoic acid also has been shown to restore intercellular glutathione. It also fights type II diabetes, helps lupus and erectile dysfunction, detoxifies heavy metals, and much more. It is found in yams, organ meats (particularly red meat), spinach, broccoli, potatoes, yeast, tomatoes, carrots, and beets, to name a few.

FISH OIL

Take 2,000 mg a day. Make sure that the oil is heavy-metal and pollution free. I prefer the brands Nordic and Arctic. Do not buy at a chain store. When it comes to fish oil, most oils are contaminated by heavy metals, and, unfortunately, with this supplement you get what you pay for.

Unless you have been living under a rock, you have probably heard by now that fish oil contains omega-3 fatty acids and that is good for you. However, a lot of people still can't tell their omega-3s from their omega-6s. Unfortunately, in modern society, we have become very scared of fats and oils. This has many ill effects on our health. (Remember, eating healthy fat will not make you fat. In fact, it will help you to maintain a healthy weight.)

Omega-3 and omega-6 are both essential fatty acids, meaning we cannot make them on our own and have to get them from our diet. In modern diets, there are few sources of omega-3 fatty acids, mainly the fat of cold-water fish, such as sardines, salmon, herring, and mackerel. They are also found in krill (a small shrimp-like crustacean, the delicacy of whales) and in grass-fed beef. Omega-3s play an important role in lowering inflammation (also in joints) and fighting cancer, depression, and weight gain. They also improve the health of your heart, bones, arteries, brain, and all cells, to name but a few benefits.

In the typical modern diet, omega-6s are everywhere. Although found in seeds and nuts, they are also found in refined vegetable oils, fast food, soy, junk food, snack food, cookies, and sweets. If it's the type of food you scarf down and feel guilty after, you can bet your bottom dollar that it contains omega-6s. Ideally, the omega-6/omega-3 ratio should be 1:1, although 2:1 or 3:1 is still acceptable. Unfortunately, a lot of people consume these fats in a ratio of 20:1 or even 50:1! This is why you must up your omega-3s and cut down on your omega-6s.

Now, I know this is not riveting stuff, but bear with me. There are two omega-3 fatty acids that our bodies *must* have: DHA (or docosahexaenoic acid) and EPA (eicosapentaenoic acid). Plant sources contain a precursor omega-3 (alpha-linolenic acid, called ALA) that the body must convert to EPA and DHA. EPA and DHA are the building blocks for hormones that control immune function, blood clotting, and cell growth as well as components of cell membranes. They are found in, for example, garbanzo beans (the beans that delicious stuff called hummus is made from) as well as nuts such as walnuts and flaxseeds.

FREEZE-DRIED ALOE VERA

Take as needed.

(For this one, I have to thank Megan, a young CRPS patient from Canada who "tested" this in the field and first told me about this). Freeze-dried aloe-vera capsules have been shown in clinical trials to effectively reduce urinary frequency, burning, and pain that are a part of many bladder disorders, but especially interstitial cystitis/painful bladder syndrome (IC/PBS) (sometimes also called prostatitis in men or chronic pelvic pain in women) that often affects patients suffering from CRPS. The Urology Wellness

Center in Rockville, Maryland, conducted a double-blind, placebo-controlled study of Desert Harvest aloe-vera capsules in IC/PBS patients. The results showed that 87.5 percent of the patients who completed the study received relief from at least some of their symptoms. Fifty percent received significant relief from all or most of their symptoms and were able to return to a more normal lifestyle. Only one patient did not respond within the first thirty days.

Patients with interstitial cystitis should be cautious about using liquid aloe vera since it is often preserved with high concentrations of citric acid, which may be irritating to the bladder. Freeze-dried aloe vera from the whole plant—with no additives, no fillers, and no heat treatment—has been proven to be the most effective type of aloe for treating interstitial cystitis, painful bladder syndrome, nonbacterial prostatitis, and chronic pelvic pain.

The theory is that the aloe plant helps IC patients in several ways. When processed correctly, the powder maintains its high levels of glycosaminoglycans (GAG). The first lining of the bladder destroyed by IC is a GAG layer. The aloe plant is also a natural anti-inflammatory, antibiotic, analgesic, and antimicrobial agent but only when used in its super-strength form.

Take 100 mg of flaxseed oil daily.

POMEGRANATE JUICE

Take 8 oz daily.

This is one of the only juices we advocate drinking. In general, juice contains massive amounts of sugar (even natural juices) that spike your blood-glucose levels and leads to cellular inflammation. Although pomegranate juice is not really a supplement, research from around the world confirms that pomegranate is one of nature's most concentrated sources of antioxidants. Pomegranate juice protects your heart, lowers blood pressure, fights cancer and aging, and most astoundingly, according to one new study, can reverse atherosclerosis,[69] something that used to be believed not to be possible.

ADRENAL SUPPORT

We recommend "High Absorption Stress & Adrenal Support" chewable tablets by New Health Products (1-800-828-1108), one tablet three times a day.

Supplements designed specifically for adrenal fatigue will nourish, strengthen, support, and optimize your adrenal function. They will also help to support homeostatic balance in the body and optimize biochemical communication in order to obtain a healthy response by these glands to stress. All eight B vitamins are essential for healthy adrenal function, as they act as catalysts in adrenal functions. Of the eight, the most important are vitamins B3 (niacin), B5 (pantothenic acid), and B6 (pyridoxine). B vitamins should be taken sublingually (dissolved in the mouth). The reason for this is that it delivers B12 directly to the bloodstream, bypassing the digestive system, which results in its maximum absorption.

METHYLFOLATE (5-METHYLTETRAHYDROFOLATE [5-MTHF])

Start by taking 400 mcg every day. You may feel slightly "odd" for three days or so, as your body has to adjust. When this feeling does not go away, start by taking 250 mcg with almond or peanut butter. When you have adjusted, add 1,000 mcg/day (you will go through an adjusting period again), repeating this process until you can tell that your energy is improved. This is your optimum dosage. You must take electrolytes and glutathione one hour prior to 5-MTHF. Drink natural electrolytes, such as coconut water with lime, or water with lime and a magnesium/calcium supplement.

> *You may also use herbal tea with lime juice. The lime juice should be freshly squeezed. Avoid folic acid–blocking drugs, such as birth control or methotrexate, drugs which increase homocysteine, such as nitrous oxide (most used in dentistry), and antacids as they block absorption of vitamin B12 and other nutrients.*

Patients who suffer from CRPS should never take folic acid or eat foods enriched with folic acid, like pasta (please see chapter 4 for information about the MTHFR gene mutation). Even if, by some slim chance, you do not suffer from this gene mutation, this is still sage advice to follow for anyone. Folic acid is synthetic and foreign to our bodies. 5-MTHF is a naturally occurring, predominant form of folate commonly found in cells and is essential for overall health, as it participates as a cofactor in a reaction that involves the remethylation of homocysteine to methionine. Unlike synthetic folic acid, 5-MTHF can be used directly by the body, without the need for an additional conversion via the enzyme 5,10-methylenetetrahydrofolate reductase (MTHFR).

MAGNESIUM (YOUR "STRESS MINERAL")

> *We recommended Natural Calm™ by Natural Vitality™, available on amazon.com (dosage as recommended by manufacturer unless directed otherwise by your health-care professional).*

Involved in pain-perception pathways and muscle contraction, magnesium may improve tenderness and pain. It is also involved in healthy brain and neurological function and bone density. Magnesium is beneficial in helping your body cope with stress and in helping you sleep. Enough said.

SELENIUM

> *I recommend taking 55 mcg of selenomethionine per day. Selenomethionine has the best bioavailability with an absorption*

rate of roughly 90 percent. It is organic and yeast free. When compared with other selenium supplements, selenomethionine proves to be the most applicable and safest for long-term therapeutic use.

Selenium is a trace element that is naturally present in many foods, such as Brazil nuts (up to seventy micrograms per nut!), liver, shellfish, and sunflower seeds, to name but a few. It is also available as a dietary supplement. Selenium is required by the body for proper functioning of the thyroid gland, for glutathione production, and for mercury detoxification. It is crucial in fighting peripheral neuropathy. It may help protect against free-radical damage, cancer, and autoimmune disease. A deficiency in selenium can lead to pain in the muscles and joints, unhealthy hair, and white spots on the fingernails.

UBIQUINOL (OR COENZYME Q10)

> *If you're over forty, Dr. Mercola highly recommends taking a reduced form of coenzyme Q10 called ubiquinol, because it's far more effectively absorbed by your body. (Ubiquinol is the reduced, electron-rich form of coenzyme Q10.)*
>
> *If you take statin (high cholesterol) drugs, it is crucial to take coenzyme Q10, since statin drugs interfere with your body's natural CoQ10 production.*
>
> *Take 150 mg twice a day for two weeks and after that 100 mg a day for the rest of your life.*

Coenzyme Q10 is almost like a vitamin, but since the body naturally makes it, it isn't called a vitamin. CoQ10 (as it is also commonly known) has been called "the single most crucial nutrient to supplement every cell in your body" by Dr. Mercola. Your cells use it to produce energy your body needs for cell growth and maintenance. Coenzymes help enzymes work to digest food and perform other body processes, and they help protect the heart and skeletal muscles.

Coenzyme Q10 also functions as an antioxidant that protects the body from damage caused by harmful molecules and therefore decreases inflammation. CoQ10 has been shown to help prevent or retard development of a fatty liver related to obesity; to fight inflammation, free-radical damage, and cancer; to protect against high blood pressure; and to help prevent heart attacks.

Last but not least, and sure to appeal to everybody's vanity, CoQ10 is an excellent tool in your antiaging arsenal. Think of this supplement as your fairy godmother, giving you a makeover from the inside out. One study in Japan found a *significant* slowing down of the aging process in a group of mice that were given Ubiquinol.[70]

CoQ10 is naturally present in small amounts in a wide variety of foods, but its levels are particularly high in organ meats, such as heart, liver, and kidney, as well as beef, sardines, mackerel, and peanuts.

ACETYL-L-CARNITINE

Take 250–500 mg a day as needed for muscle pain. Although most people do not need extra L-carnitine, people who suffer from CRPS may benefit from supplementation. Vegetarians may also need to supplement. It is best taken in its activated form.

L-carnitine is an amino acid that is directly involved in cellular fatty-acid metabolism. Although it can be obtained from your diet (red meats are a particularly rich source), it is also produced in your liver and kidneys. Most of the carnitine in your body is stored in your muscles and heart, where it is needed to transfer fatty acids into mitochondria so they can be oxidized for energy. An L-carnitine deficiency may cause muscle pain due to inefficient cellular-energy metabolism (mitochondrial myopathy), and L-carnitine has been shown to be effective for nerve pain in some cases. L-carnitine has also been shown to improve mental clarity and overall energy and to fight aging, type II diabetes, and cancer.

D-RIBOSE

Take 500 mg three times a day for four weeks and 500 mg twice a day after as needed.

This may be the most important supplement in your CRPS and chronic-fatigue arsenal. D-ribose is a naturally occurring sugar that has been shown to support the production and recycling of ATP (think of it as fuel for your car), which helps to increase energy production in stressed tissues. It may even be effective to alleviate migraines, a symptom often suffered by CRPS patients.

MALIC ACID

It is most effective when combined with magnesium.
Start at a daily recommended dosage of 600 mg twice a day coupled with 150 mg of magnesium twice per day, and slowly increase your levels to 1,200 mg of malic acid twice per day coupled with 300 mg of magnesium, also twice per day, over 2–3 months.

Malic acid is an organic acid made by all living organisms. It is also responsible for that pleasantly sour tang in apples and other fruits, and it is sometimes referred to as "fruit acid." Malic acid is involved in energy production in muscle cells. It is necessary for glucose metabolism, which is important for nourishing muscles and nerves. Malic acid increases ATP production (cellular fuel). It will enhance your mood and may help reduce muscle discomfort and overall pain in those who suffer from CRPS.

CURCUMIN

Take 300 mg a day. It is contraindicated for those on blood-thinning medications or those with gall-bladder disease.

Curcumin is the key component of turmeric, and it is responsible for the spice's distinctive mustard-yellow color. This spice is popular in the Far East, especially in curry-spice blends. It's a member of the ginger family and comes from a root just like ginger. Curcumin is a proven antioxidant and a powerful anti-inflammatory. Some research shows it can even boost your immunity, may show benefits in fighting cancer, and is a powerful antiviral. It has also shown benefits in helping to relieve the symptoms of irritable bowel syndrome (IBS) as well as arthritis and menstrual cramps. It also positively affects nerve pain.

ZINC

Take 220 mg twice per day. Taking zinc together with vitamin C may cause nausea.

Zinc is an essential mineral that is naturally present in some foods such as oysters, crabs, wheat germ, pumpkin seeds, watermelon seeds, roast beef, dark chocolate and cocoa powder, lamb, and peanuts.

Zinc is required by your body for maintaining a sense of smell, keeping a healthy immune system, building proteins, triggering enzymes, tissue growth and repair, skin health, and making DNA. Zinc also helps the cells in your body communicate by functioning as a neurotransmitter. A deficiency in zinc can lead to stunted growth, diarrhea, impotence, hair loss, eye and skin lesions, impaired appetite, and depressed immunity. In addition, taking extra zinc during pregnancy has been shown to be much more effective at preventing stretch marks than rubbing oil or lotion on your tummy.

Please note that *too* much zinc may cause nausea, vomiting, and diarrhea. If you experience these side effects, please back off your dosage.

13

Tales from the War Front: Real Patient Stories

Temper us in fire, and we grow stronger. When we suffer, we survive.

—C. Clare

No one can tell what goes on in between the person you were and the person you become. No one can chart that blue and lonely section of hell. There are no maps of the change. You just come out the other side.

—S. King

I have asked a few of my patients to tell their stories here. I did not give them a specific format to use, as I wanted each patient to tell it from the heart. I wish I could write a whole book filled with my patient's stories, as each one is a monument to a battle hard fought and won. I owe all my patients a wealth of gratitude, for as they learned from me, I learned from them.

CARLOS JASSO'S STORY

I consider Carlos to be my "Patient Zero." Not only was he the first patient to complete treatment, but it was while treating him that

Putting Out the Fire

I discovered the power of Frequency Specific Microcurrent when combined with reconnecting the vagus-nerve communication. Carlos first came in as white as a sheet. He was obviously in severe pain, and he was giving up. With him was his nine-month old baby son and lovely wife, Tanya. I looked at his baby, and I knew that I could not fail. It wasn't an option. Today, Carlos is living a normal life. He is now a youth pastor and is taking trips to exotic places, such as Africa, as part of his mission work. He is pain free and has undergone abdominal surgery after completing treatment, without any complications.

Hello, my name is Carlos Jasso, and I have full-body RSD. Unlike the normal effects of RSD (affecting a limb), mine was internal. You see, my RSD started in the internal abdominal area in 2005 before it spread to my full body within a month after being diagnosed in 2007. Yes, it took two years before I was diagnosed. Once diagnosed I tried an electric TENS unit temporarily, and that is how the RSD rapidly spread to my full body within a week of using it. (Be careful on the methods chosen to treat yourself; some do not help and can actually make you worse.)

My primary doctor no longer could help me with my pain, and I was sent to a pain specialist where I was given the maximum amounts of pain medication, such as morphine and other opioids, and many more. Along with the medications, I was administered spinal injections, five in one visit each time I was seen. None of it would truly take the pain away. I was told by numerous doctors that I was on enough narcotics to kill thirty full-grown mules or a hundred full-grown men. Even with all that, all it was doing was allowing me to go through life feeling like a zombie, yet it wasn't stopping the raging tornado inside of me. As time went on, I fought to keep going on, when it actually got worse. In 2009–10 it started affecting my ability to eat or drink anything, as a simple bite of food or drink of water would have an excruciating effect. After ingesting food or liquid, the pain would literally drop me to the floor in the fetal position and tears would flow as the severity level of the pain was unlike anything I've ever felt. I had arrived at a place where I wouldn't eat or drink anything because of the fear of the pain RSD was causing to my body.

It was then that a dear friend of ours had attended a seminar that Dr. Katina was speaking at, and she called and asked if she could share my problem with her. After that, we decided to go see Dr. Katinka. I will admit I truly had my doubts and was very skeptical that there would be help in this, but it beat the alternatives of causing even more trauma against my body to try and correct an injury caused by trauma in the first place. I don't understand that logic at all. Well my wife, Tanya, and I went to see if this doctor could actually help me. We sat and spoke with Dr. Katinka, and she asked what I knew about RSD. I shared all the knowledge I had about this rare disorder. We then tried a treatment, and Dr. Katinka asked if we would do her a favor. She asked me to do the one thing I was starting to fear, and she asked if I would go and try to eat something and then come back to her office.

I recall making a comment to my wife I don't know about this, but nonetheless we did, and for the first time in six months, I could eat and did not have any pain! I believe that is when I realized how badly my body was starving itself. I had disconnected from food, because I had to. I then started seeing Dr. Katinka ten times a week for twelve weeks as my wife worked about fifteen minutes away from Dr. Katinka's office. There was a great improvement as I was undergoing treatment, but then my progress seemed to stall, and the pain was returning. This was around week eight, as I recall.

Dr. Katinka was determined, however, and was not going to give in to this monster and called in help. I was then used to test for a frequency from a device that her patients now know as Frequency Specific Microcurrent. The help of these two techniques that Dr. Katinka used helped me gain life back. By week ten I was off all medications. For the first time since 2005, I was pain free on some days. Then, as the treatment progressed, the soreness became less and the pain-free days more. I've not had a treatment in almost four years, and I am still pain free. No burning, stabbing, sharp shooting, sensitivity to light or air, nor extremely bad migraines. I am now living without fear of pain, and I am not using any medications. I have become a pastor and now travel to other nations. Dr. Katinka van Der Merwe was a godsent blessing to help me fight against the beast of pain. Over time, she has become the tool of healing many lives. She is my guardian angel against this beast. And I am so thankful for all she has done. Dr. Katinka gave me back my life when everyone else had given up on me.

DAVID SMITH'S STORY

> David started care in my office in late 2015. He is now under maintenance care. David and his wife, Deb, are wonderful people whom I simply adore. David calls me "ma'am" and often brings me his homemade jams, which are really an art form. I am addicted especially to his strawberry jam, as he has miraculously figured out how to pack one pound of strawberries into a tiny mason jar of jam. David will tell you that he is an "old Baptist minister" and he has frequently sat down with new CRPS patients in my office and offered to pray for them. He is also a black belt in karate who can still hold his own, no matter the age of his opponent. I consider myself the lucky one for meeting him. David's story is told by his wonderful wife, Deb.

HOW IT ALL STARTED

In preparation for retirement, David finally decided to have corrective surgery on his right foot to relieve two painful conditions, a hammertoe on his big toe and a bunionectomy on the side of the same toe. The toe was straightened and an implant and screw placed to keep the toe straight. A second implant was placed in the toe next to it as it was also beginning to develop hammertoe. The stabbing pain emerged not long after surgery, so nerve relaxers and strong pain medications and antidepressants were prescribed. After a few months, a second surgery was performed, this time on the ball of the foot as the surgeon thought that a nerve had attached to scar tissue, but the pain persisted. He was in PT three days a week. As the pain level intensified and became more frequent, I remembered my sister-in-law describing similar pain after a surgery on her hand several years ago that was diagnosed quickly as RSD. When I asked David's surgeon if it could be RSD, he looked at me with a dreaded look on his face and said, "Oh God, I hope not."

We were referred to a neurologist who confirmed RSD. He took over pain-management medications and saw David on a monthly basis. The pain and drugs overtook David's life. I continued intense research to learn about any successful treatments. That's when it really got scary. I heard of a pain specialist about eighty miles from us and made an appointment. David had three nerve blocks that provided temporary relief, but for a shorter time with each injection. She then managed his orders for more physical therapy, specific for RSD, and referred him to a cardiologist for a stress test and EKG to clear him to receive a channel-blocking medication.

THE MEDS

David's prescriptions have included morphine, OxyContin, Lyrica, Cymbalta, clonazepam, cyclobenzaprine, clonidine patches, butorphanol, hydromorphone, meloxicam, Norvasc, zolpidem, and a compounding pharmacy cream that was very expensive. The medications were his temporary relief from pain, but his life was about limiting activities and never committing to anything, since pain controlled his life and he couldn't think or function well under the influence of the pain meds he had to take in order to survive it.

THE FINANCIAL BLESSINGS AND CHALLENGES

David's short-term disability paid 50 percent of his base salary for six months. I was working thirty-two-plus hours per week in the front office for a dentist. David had paid premiums for years for a long-term disability plan through his employer that paid 80 percent of his base salary after short-term disability ended, payable to age sixty-seven so long as you remained disabled. That company provided us with an agency that began the process of filing for disability under Social Security. They secured full disability in six months.

When we received back pay, the long term–disability insurance company recovered most of what they had paid us and began paying the difference between the SSDI benefit and the amount they would have been paying.

A few months later, they advised us that benefit would end unless we could prove he was still unable to work. We appealed it, and they paid a lump sum back pay for those months but removed his future benefit unless we appealed again. They had a doctor in Houston who decided he could be a batch clerk. I was exhausted with them and didn't have the stamina it would take to prepare another appeal for the small amount they would pay. I had spent countless hours on the phone and gathering documents from his doctors and physical-therapist records and preparing the narrative for the appeal.

Our company health insurance remained in effect for a year, and then we went under Healthcare Marketplace coverage. David became eligible for Medicare after two years on disability.

THE MENTAL AND EMOTIONAL FALLOUT

While his pain was topping the charts more frequently and his medication levels increased, other symptoms of the condition included fatigue, deepening depression, hopelessness, withdrawal from any social commitments, embarrassment of being unable to stop tears rolling down his face during severe pain attacks, and living with a fear that each step would result in a pain event. I'd brought a chair to him many times when a step caused the stabbing pain and he could not walk further. Life as we had known it ceased. The plans for enjoying retirement were pushed to the back of our minds, ignored so as not to bring further emotional pain.

HOPE LOST

I spent countless hours searching every website for any successful treatments I could find for RSD, and I learned through RSD Hope of a clinical trial for neridronate infusion that seemed hopeful with one of the sites within driving distance. Few had signed up, and they feared the study location might be canceled. Knowing many people who suffer from RSD made me post about the study to the Power Over Pain support group chapter in my state, their leader and I began a dialogue.

In preparation for David's first infusion, we carefully made sure his pain stayed under control the day before, reporting a pain level of three. When we got to the site, we were reminded that he would have had to have a higher pain level the previous day to enter the study. We and everyone at the center cried. Even the director's efforts to get reentry to the study at a later date were unsuccessful. We were devastated. Our faith was tested. Why? Why? Why? Why would this happen when we were so close to possible relief ? I can't even describe what driving back home was like. We believe everything happens for a purpose, but this one was about too much to handle.

After that, we were referred to another pain specialist. He was going to do a different form of nerve block. He would sedate David in order to do the procedure and would need a blood and urine test. They would let us know when the procedure would be done. We drove eighty miles, we waited two hours to see him, and he acted like we shouldn't have had any explanations or questions about what was best. The next call we received was to set up his follow-up. Duh! When insurance retrieved their payment, we still ended up with a bill of about $600. Live and learn!

NEVER, EVER, GIVE UP!
With a passion to help others as well as herself, my Power Over Pain dearest friend contacted me a few months later about a doctor she was hearing about who seemed to have some amazing results helping RSD patients. I began my research into the work of Dr. Katinka van der Merwe of the Neurologic Relief Center in Fayetteville, Arkansas. I left a message on the voice mail. I was shocked when my phone rang around seven or eight o'clock that Friday evening and the caller was Dr. van der Merwe! She described the treatment plan she follows for RSD treatment, advising

that she would be able to tell us within a couple of weeks if her treatments would be helpful to him. She stated that there is no cure for RSD but her treatments do not involve medications, injections, or any invasive treatment. I asked if she thought other patients might be willing to speak with me about their experiences and progress under her treatment, and she gave me several names of people from around the United States, explaining that most of her patients came from outside Arkansas for RSD treatment. I contacted two. They shared their amazing stories of treatment and relief from the high pain levels and highly recommended we try to see if David could be helped. I spoke with my boss, advising that I felt we had to try and that I understood that my job would need to be filled with a replacement if we stayed for several weeks of treatment. He told me to go for the initial two weeks and then we would discuss what to do about my position.

THE CONSULT

Some of the pain triggers of RSD include physical, mental, and emotional stress. David was a little nervous during the consult, and his foot began to swell, a surefire indicator that the pain would shortly follow. He asked if he could remove his shoe, and a few minutes later, he asked to take one of his pain pills. Dr. van der Merwe said removing the shoe was absolutely fine, but her response to taking the pain med was to ask if he could wait a few minutes. She then had him lie down and asked him to rate his pain level, and he reported it was increasing and at about a 3 out of 10 on the pain scale. She placed a finger on each side of his neck below and behind his ears, and she began to explain that her treatments address the central nervous system.

About a minute or so later, she asked his pain level, and it was coming down and about two. We were shocked! It *never* ceased without drugs! Another couple of minutes passed when she asked again what his pain level was, and his reply was, "Ma'am, it's at zero!" She explained that it would probably return but that the treatment plan she follows does result in long-term relief for many patients. We set up the appointments for the following day and went to an extended stay hotel to begin another journey to find relief.

AN UNEXPECTED BENEFIT

A blessing and great help has been an amazing support group of others with RSD being treated by Dr. Katinka. For the first time, David met and talked with others who have the same pain and other symptoms associated with RSD. It brought great comfort to all of them to share their stories and weird symptoms with each other. We found a RSD "family" who socialized and supported and cheered David on for every step of progress. We will always be there for each other to pray for, uplift, celebrate, and encourage each other.

RESULTS

At this writing, it's been about nine months since our first visit to Dr. Katinka. Her approach totally makes sense. RSD/CRPS is *nerve* pain, so why not treat the central nervous system directly? Drugs dull the pain, can be addictive, leave you unable to function or think clearly, are expensive, and have many bad side effects. David's response to treatment set a record as the fastest-responding patient to treatment. He's had only one light short pain event. Before and during treatment, we continue to deal with an emotionally difficult situation that has taken a great toll. Every single day is a mental and emotional struggle. I'm amazed that he remains free of pain. He has RSD, and there is no cure.

We see a lot of continuing improvements, such as a lessening of the frequency and severity of the flu-like symptoms that occasionally just come over him. He has to pay attention to his body as a "buzzing" sensation in his foot feels like a warning that it is going to start swelling. He requires sleep to "rejuvenate" and starts each day waking up in what he describes as "brain fog," an inability to think clearly for about thirty minutes to an hour. We believe in the power of prayer, and we have many who have been faithful to pray for David and can see God's hand over us in many ways. We can deal with these remaining symptoms, even as annoying as they are. We will take each day as it comes, pray for a cure, and keep Dr. Katinka van der Merwe on our speed dial! The awesome team at The Neurologic Relief Center are second to none. They have a heart for those who hurt. There is a family atmosphere that celebrates every improvement for every patient. May God bless them.

BRENDA'S STORY

> *Brenda was one of the very first patients suffering from CRPS whom I treated. Brenda lives in Tennessee with her husband and has been in remission for nearly five years now. When I met Brenda, she was no longer able to work. Today, she owns a restaurant with her husband in which she works. She is on her feet all day long almost daily. On a very bad day, her pain will reach about a 2/10 on the pain scale.*

My story started with me having a heel spur removed from my right foot in December of 2009. Two weeks after the surgery, I was able to remove my boot, but after the very first step I took, I knew something was not right. I was in more pain than before the surgery. How could this be? The doctor told me to give it some time and come back in two weeks. Two weeks passed, and the pain was worse. I had sharp, shooting pain, swelling, and burning in my right foot; my foot was always cold and always hurt. I went back, in more pain than before the surgery. My doctor didn't know what the problem could be.

After weeks of going back and forth, I went to another doctor, and thus my two-year journey began, going to doctor after doctor after doctor. I had one put me in a cast just to see if it would help because he just didn't know what to do. I became so frustrated, not being able to work, not being able to do the things I used to do; even little things seemed so hard to do. By now I was on long-term disability, and I was thinking, "What will happen if I can never go back to work? I won't be able to help my husband financially." I didn't know what to do!

Finally, I went to see a neurologist, who listened to my story and checked the medical records I had brought from all the doctors I had seen. He went out of the office, came back in, looked at my foot, and said, "I believe you have chronic pain syndrome or reflex sympathetic dystrophy (RSD)." He then told me it's a neurological condition with the nerves overfiring. I felt a lump in my throat and tears welling up in my eyes. I was just so thankful that someone had finally found out what was wrong. After two years, I had finally been diagnosed. Even though he did tell me there was not much they could do for this and I would have it the rest of my life, I was just so thankful to finally have a name for whatever was wrong. I felt like no one believed me; I had people ask me, "How are you doing today? You look good, you're walking around—you must be OK."

The one person who always seemed to understand and believe me was my husband, who, by the way, has been incredible through all this. Not many are as lucky as I am with their spouse believing them about the pain. I have met so many people with this disease and still their families don't believe them. People think, because they can't see anything wrong with you, that there is nothing wrong. RSD is a monster of a disease. It robs you of your life. It makes you think you're crazy.

After being diagnosed with RSD, I began to see a pain-management doctor. He started me on lots of medications, none of which worked. I went and had nerve blocks every week for about three to four months. They were a waste of time and money. I had to drive about two hours every week to have this done, and it just was not helping. I went to my next appointment with my pain-management doctor and told him that the nerve blocks and medications did not help. He said, "We can try you on the stimulator that they insert into your back." As soon as they said that, I wanted to run. I knew I was not letting anyone cut into me again. Surgery was what started my RSD, and I was not having anyone cut into me. I had read that once you have RSD, it could spread, especially to a new surgery site. I had to figure something out, and I had to be fast.

I had been on Facebook one day and saw an ad for a teleconference for RSD. I mentioned it to my husband, and we decided to sign up to listen. This doctor was saying she could possibly tell within the first ten minutes of the treatment if she would be able to help me, which I thought was too good to be true. Really? Ten minutes? I thought this sounded too good to be true. But what did I have to lose? If I went there and it didn't help, I'd leave. Just gas money spent. If I did get relief, I would consider staying for treatment.

My husband and I talked it over for a little while, thinking that if I didn't go I could be missing out on getting relief and getting my life back. We decided I was going. I called and talked to the doctor's assistant. She was so friendly, and she set us up with an appointment. We drove to Fayetteville, Arkansas, from Springville, Tennessee.

When we walked into her office, we were surprised by how friendly everyone was. Dr. Katinka talked privately with my husband and myself and then ordered X-rays and a test to see where my problem spots were. I then came back later that afternoon and was called to Dr. Katinka's table. She started to tell me what she would be doing and explained every step. She had asked what pain level I was at, and I had told her about an eight; then she started the treatment and was able to get me down to about a two. I started to feel less pain, less burning. This is not possible, I thought. Was this my imagination?

I stayed at the hotel for a month, receiving treatments every day. After a month I was to go home for a month and then return for another month of treatments. After about three weeks at home, the pain started up again. Pat, my husband, called Dr. Katinka and told her what was going on. She said I needed to get back there as soon as possible. The longer I was gone, the harder it would be to get the pain under control. We left shortly after that, and I began another month of treatment.

I can remember that one time, when Pat came to visit me, I was walking after a treatment, and the ladies in the office said he had become emotional because I was walking without pain. I was walking! I hadn't done that much before the treatments. During treatment I began to take myself off my medications, as I wanted to be sure they were not masking anything. I had to know if the treatments were really working. I was eating healthier and noticed I was losing weight. I was able to do more walking than I was in the past without pain.

I could not believe how I was feeling. I felt like I was getting my life back. It was amazing. I had begun to miss my family dearly and wanted to go home. I was about done with my month and was getting excited to see everyone. I missed my home with my husband, my children, and my grandchildren. It was time for me to leave after my second month. I knew I would miss Dr. Katinka and her amazing staff. They are more like friends now. I had met so many wonderful people who were patients and became friends; we shared a bond because of our chronic pain.

Dr. Katinka is an amazing person and an amazing doctor. I am so grateful to her for everything she has done for me. She has given me my life back. I wish that every RSD patient could see her. I wish they too could feel as good as I do. Yes, there are days I get pain and burning, but it always calms down. It is nothing like it was before. Here I am writing this today and having a pain-free day. Thank you, Dr. Katinka.

BARBARA WALL'S STORY

Barbara started care in our office late in 2015. Prior to that, she suffered from CRPS for ten years. Barbara is one of two administrators of a fabulous CRPS support group here in Little Rock. She is one dynamic lady. Before she became sick, she was a cardiac nurse. After she got sick, she has supported and helped countless patients with CRPS navigate their care, even though she was hurting daily herself. She also organized a very successful fundraiser with her corporate experience, in order to collect money for CRPS research. As a result of her experience with CRPS and subsequent treatment in our office, her lovely daughter, Lauren, is starting school in September 2016 in order to train in this work. Barbara is currently still receiving maintenance care in our office, although not often.

Putting Out the Fire

Before I got RSD, I was living life and enjoying all things around me. I did not feel that I took much of anything for granted. In 2005, I suffered a severe injury to my cervical spine (broken neck) as well as other injuries. As if dealing with a broken neck was not enough, I received the diagnosis of reflex sympathetic dystrophy (RSD), today known as complex regional pain syndrome (CRPS). I had the opportunity to practice as a registered nurse for twenty-five years. I was hoping to get beyond this illness and the acute daily pain in order to continue my professional career. I did absolutely everything the doctors ordered and pushed myself each and every day during physical therapy. After a host of medication changes and numerous stellate ganglion blocks, lumbar sympathetic blocks, and cervical epidural steroid injections, my body did not go into remission. I was forced to quit a career I absolutely loved and began focusing on my health. Every day was full of appointments, disappointments, physical therapy, occupational and pool therapy.

I was able to establish a great team of medical doctors and felt comfortable with my care. The pain continued to overwhelm my mind and body. My family remained so supportive and encouraging, but I needed a strength so far greater than they could give. Each day was such a challenge, but with God, family, and my own inner strength, I was able to wake up every morning and tell myself, "I can, and I will do this." As days, months, and years passed by with constant pain, I was able to keep my attitude in the game of life and continue to fight this fight. I was finally approved for a spinal cord stimulator (SCS) and responded well to the three-day trial. Months after the trial, I was approved for a permanently implanted SCS. My quality of life was drastically improved, and it gave me enough relief most days to continue my daily regime of physical therapy and two hours of pool therapy. We could not decrease any of my medication, or I would have a setback. I totally relied on my SCS for pain control because I did not respond to narcotic medications.

I would define the past ten years with full-body RSD as mind blowing, traumatic, overwhelming, and most of all changing. I have a great joy for life and all the wonderful opportunities it has to offer. Opportunities are not without work, and living with this condition is work, hard work.

In June 2015, things would again change. Even though I continued to live with daily pain, that would also change. Yes, it changed for the worse. I made a simple movement with my neck and felt a horrible pop with lightning pain. I could not raise my head, and the pain was intense. My SCS would not touch the pain, which was unusual. After weeks of sleeplessness nights, severe pain, and diagnostic tests, we found the culprit. I had damaged two of the discs in my neck and therefore pushed my SCS paddle to the right. Because the paddle had shifted, I lost all coverage for pain on the left side. Now I had to decide what to do and how to treat this. My concerns were so overwhelming about surgery and the risk of exacerbating the RSD. My spine specialist was also concerned about the surgery and the risks involved. We did not want to send my body into a state that would push me back to the initial insult. I did not want to *ever* go back to where I was ten years ago. I have dedicated my life to rehabilitation and maintaining what I have achieved with all of my therapies.

After lots of research and answers to many prayers, I found a doctor in my home state of Arkansas who was having amazing results with RSD patients. Dr. Katinka van der Merwe is a chiropractor who specializes in restoring balance to the autonomic nervous system. October 12, 2015, was my first appointment with Dr. Katinka, and I was cautiously optimistic. I had never been evaluated nor treated by a chiropractor before. She does not perform manipulations as part of her "Three Punch" system. The treatment modalities and techniques that she uses are unlike any I have ever received. Her technique is painless, noninvasive, and does not require any medications. The day I arrived at her clinic, my pain level was 8/10. After my initial evaluation and treatment, my pain had dropped to a 4/10. As the weeks and treatments progressed, my pain level has remained at a zero the majority of the time.

As most of you are aware, RSD has no known cure, but there is hope in hopeless situations. Even with my continued spine issues and the need for surgery on my cervical spine, I have been able to maintain low to no pain with my RSD. I cannot tell you how amazing it is after ten years of chronic pain to actually sleep throughout the night, to not feel like you are burning from within, and to finally be able to plan events in my life.

After completing ten weeks of treatments with Dr. Katinka, I have been able to slowly stop all of my RSD prescription medications. My mind feels so much more alert, and the ability to communicate without losing your train of thought is amazing. I am forever grateful that Dr. Katinka has such a passion and desire to help those who suffer from this isolating, devastating, life-altering condition. Do not accept life as it is if you are suffering, and never give up hope! I encourage you to be your own advocate and to get help.

14

Don't. You. Ever. Stop. Fighting.

To disprove the theory that all crows are black, you only need to find one white crow.

—Professor William James, Harvard

Never give in. Never give in. Never, never, never, never—in nothing, great or small, large or petty—never give in, except to convictions of honor and good sense. Never yield to force. Never yield to the apparently overwhelming might of the enemy.

—Winston Churchill

Personally, I believe that every single thing happens for a reason, large or small. Four weeks ago, I had a brutal glimpse (mind you, just a *glimpse*) into the hell that CRPS patients go through. While I have always been very caring and sympathetic toward my patients, I could not truly begin to understand what you guys go through. As I mentioned early in this book, I have always been very healthy. However, shortly after giving birth, I started experiencing sharp shooting pains in my left eye. Blaming it on having my glasses adjusted, I thought it would go away, just like every other single symptom or illness I have ever had. The next day, the pain had progressed into my entire left face, and it started to resemble nerve pain in every way. As the pain progressed down my face, it started to resemble acute trigeminal neuralgia in a frightening way, which, like CRPS, is known as a "suicide disease."

I could not accept this self-diagnosis, however. After many days, I convinced myself that it was simply tooth related. Desperate, I went to my dentist with whom I have a great working relationship. "Please," I begged him. "Just tell me what is *causing* it." After he studied my X-rays and did my exam, he said the words I have secretly been dreading: "it's definitely not your teeth."

I would like to say that I left his office with a plan, but I had none. I was freaking out. I remember thinking, "Oh my God. Is this what my patients go through every day?" Every night, the pain intensified. Somehow it was worse at night. It didn't help that my new baby was awake during the worst of it, as he still had his nights and days confused. Desperate, I wanted pain relief any way I could get it. Tequila? Hydrocodone? Bring it on! Now, this was *me*, the same person who gave natural birth three times, who never takes medication no matter what. Unfortunately for me, I was breastfeeding, and numbing was not an option. The pain was horrific not only in its intensity but also in its relentlessness. I knew enough to frighten me, enough to not go and seek a diagnosis after seeing endless specialists. I knew what my options would be in any case. Desperate, after crying on my dad's table one day, his calm voice of reason finally got through to me. Fear was controlling me. I decided to get back to what I knew. I focused on my treatment instead of finding a diagnosis and in *believing* that it could and *would* get better. And so it did. Not because I willed it, but because I was incredibly blessed, had great doctors to work on me, and because I did not suffer from CRPS, although I did suffer from nerve pain.

It is an experience that I will always treasure in a weird way. The pain left just enough of a mark to make me a better doctor. The hardest thing was having hope, even after such a short time. Panic is a nasty beast that nips away at you, especially when it is dark and people (with no pain) are sleeping around you. I cannot imagine what you must feel like, when everyone tells you, (all the greatest doctors in the world), that you will suffer forever and that there is no cure.

I wish I could count the times that I have been hotly reprimanded and debated at lectures, online, or in my practice, by people suffering from CRPS. Basically, they all say the same thing: "But there is no cure for CRPS! Who are you to say it could get better? Are you smarter than all these experts and researchers and doctors?" To this, I like to quote my father, who often uses a quote by a professor from Harvard named William Jones: "To disprove the theory that all crows are black, you only need to find one white crow." I have seen people suffering from CRPS find their way back to health. I have seen a white crow.

This is an extremely subjective and sensitive topic. When the word "cure" is used, that brings to mind visions of a miracle pill, injection, or surgery studied and proven by perhaps a promising double-blind study and excitedly announced by the media. Please believe me when I tell you that it probably won't happen that way. The failure in finding such a "cure" lies in the theory of what CRPS is or what it is caused by. It is a complex problem, not a puzzle with a single solution. It is not a condition that can be healed by a miracle chemical; it is a body where a whole bunch of things went wrong.

CRPS must be approached by a method where every system involved is checked and rebuilt, if necessary, in a systematic way. I've personally known numerous patients and acquaintances who consider themselves healed from the neurologic symptoms of CRPS. I have heard people tell their stories about finding their own recoveries in their own ways on the Internet. I have seen it with my own eyes, and I have seen these patients stay better. If even one patient can do it, why can't your body?

The number-one thing all successful patients have in common is hope. Hope allows patients to still try and to do what they have to do in order to get better. It has been said that a sign of insanity is doing the same thing over and over, expecting a different outcome. If you are sick today, it is clear that what you have been doing up to now is not working and that it is time to approach your condition differently. When patients assume responsibility for their own health-care challenges, do their own research, and are willing to do what it takes, they *can* make dramatic improvements. If you suffer a great deal, which is true for most people with CRPS, even long-term decrease of your pain by 30 percent will be a massive relief, and it means that the quality of your life will vastly improve. Never ever give up.

WHAT YOU FOCUS ON EXPANDS

Let's pretend that you are healthy, and one day, while sitting around, you get the crazy idea to complete a marathon. Let's say you are not a runner and frankly a bit of a couch potato. What would you guess is the best way to start? I'd say, turn to Google. That is my first step these days. Do you Google "ten reasons that most people will never finish a marathon"? No! You go and look for tips. Advice. You follow other people who have finished marathons. Perhaps you get a coach—someone who has experience and comes highly recommended, since he or she has coached other people from the couch over the finish line. You get my drift.

> **What you give time, energy, and focus to will grow in your life. Please keep the goal of recovering alive in your heart and mind. It has been done by others. It could be done by you. Do not allow negative people around you if you can help it. Minimize the input of those you can't avoid.**

Always be on the lookout for stories of recovery; you never know what you can learn, although it is more than understandable that you may be tired and be tempted to accept the opinion that CRPS is a life sentence. Always work toward the goal to do everything in your power to help your body function at its maximum potential. This includes your diet, supplementation, and your mind-set. Even small changes add up, if these changes are made so that they become habits, as consistent as possible given your circumstances.

REPEAT AFTER ME: DOCTORS WORK FOR YOU, NOT THE OTHER WAY AROUND

As difficult as CRPS makes your life, the very least you deserve is a doctor who understands your condition and who *believes* you. I always say that CRPS patients should have the equivalent of a NASCAR pit crew on their side. Have you ever seen how the driver pulls in and they can change a tire in seconds? Every crew member knows his or her job. Every member is focused and knows what the other member is doing. Now, I am not naive. Since most doctors are not taught about CRPS in school (save for maybe a brief mention), this may be incredibly hard to find. Also, since CRPS is relatively rare, you cannot expect that your doctor should be an expert on this condition right from the start. What you can reasonably expect, however, is that your doctor becomes knowledgeable about CRPS if you choose to employ him or her as your primary-care physician. If he or she is your doctor, that person should have at least a basic understanding of the condition you are suffering from.

The first thing you must do is *your* due diligence. It starts with the basic understanding that your doctor is, in fact, employed by *you*, not the other way around. The following is so important that I am repeating it. Your doctor needs to be well informed, willing to listen, and keeping an open mind. Like we said earlier in this book, if your doctor has the nerve or audacity in this day and age, with all the research available to him or her, to tell you that the pain you suffer from is all in your head, for heaven's sake, fire the doctor. There is no excuse for that. It is not your job to convince the doctor that you are not lying, looking for attention or to score drugs, or unwell psychologically.

You have a wonderful resource in the form of the Internet. If your doctor is unsuitable to help you for whatever reason, ask other CRPS patients in your state where to turn. Please understand that this may mean that you have to travel great distances in order to find a doctor who understands CRPS. If this is at all financially possible for you, do it. Your health is worth it, and your health is *your* responsibility at the end of the day. While I understand that many people who suffer from CRPS have been wiped out financially, I do want to mention that if you have the resources, you will sometimes have to spend out of your pocket to find the best doctors or treatments. This may be the case even if your case (for instance) is a workman's comp case, you are a Medicare patient, or you live in a country with universal health care, such as Canada.

If this is a luxury you cannot afford, you still have one more option: find a good doctor who cares, and educate him or her. A lot of doctors are open to learning. Since most doctors are left brained (meaning, they use the logical part of their brain, like engineers do, for instance), they respond well to facts. Also, keep in mind that doctors do tend to be busy and overworked. For this reason, it would be best if you take them research articles about CRPS that pertain to your goals. Print this material, and hand it to them; do not ask them to look up a website, article, or link. If your doctor is unwilling to look at the material you give him or her (I'm assuming here that you are not handing your doctor piles of it during every visit), it's time to find a new doctor. Ditto if your doctor seems to think that you are faking or says completely incorrect things to you, such as that CRPS cannot spread or cannot affect the entire body. Think of you and your doctor as a team with a common goal: to make your life better. This also requires you to stay very informed and be aware of all the latest new research.

WHAT DOES REMISSION LOOK LIKE?

When patients who suffer from CRPS dream about remission, they picture themselves back in the life that they used to have before CRPS. They picture themselves "cured," having no pain ever. The truth is more complicated. You have to remember that CRPS is not like lightning that strikes unlucky, healthy people. CRPS affects those who, for whatever reason, have unhealthy nervous systems or unlucky genetics. While it is possible to compensate for your genetics, this does mean that you will have to live more carefully than most; however, it does not mean that you have to wrap yourself in figurative bubble wrap, living in fear of every bump and fall. I have had many patients, after completing their treatment, suffer injuries or undergo surgeries, with no ill effects. CRPS attacks weak spots in the nervous system if it is unable to self-limit the inflammatory cycle. A body that is functioning correctly can switch off inflammation when it is no longer appropriate.

There is a big difference between living diligently and living in fear. Living in fear means that anything can "get" you, at any time, like a predator stalking you in the bushes. You are constantly aware that it is always close by, ready to pounce. It means you are a victim, with no control. Living diligently means that you are respectful of your health, as you have seen the damage that ill health can wreck on your life, your psyche, and your loved ones. It means that you make daily choices that are most likely to result in better health. It means that you are in control. Special care must be taken during times of great stress, such as the death of a loved one, illnesses, or injuries. Think of your body as a building with a roof that has been repaired. During a monsoon, you need to be extra diligent. Do not ignore any "leaks" of energy.

Not all patients will become 100 percent pain free. However, the pain should be much more manageable, without the use of daily narcotics. Remission essentially is a process by which you regain trust in your own body's ability to heal from within. Ideally, it involves a basic understanding of why and how you got sick in the first place so that you feel more in control of your future health, rather than like a sitting duck.

CHARACTERISTICS OF HEALING

In my experience, when patients fantasize what healing will look like, it generally resembles a smooth road without many obstacles in which everyone lives happily ever after. In these fantasies of Nirvana, there are no drawbacks, healing happens fast (hence the word "cure"), and something brings about this healing from the outside in (a magical procedure, surgery, or drug). The reality is much different. For this reason, I thought it would be valuable to share the characteristics of healing that I have observed over time.

1. **Healing is hard, hard work.**
   While healing can be extremely rewarding, exciting, and fun, it also involves incredibly hard work. Besides the initial work when researching treatments as well as the practical problems you will have to sort out (financing, lodging, etc.), the actual process of healing can be very challenging. Essentially, you are signing up for a roller-coaster ride of ups and downs as well as rapid changes that all will require that you have to adapt. Your medications will have to be adjusted by a professional, and you may go through withdrawals and detoxification reactions. In addition, you will have to learn what your new boundaries are. While you may soon feel like a butterfly emerging out of a cocoon, ready to spread your wings, your nervous system more resembles a newborn fawn, vulnerable and shaky at first as it acclimates. For this reason, I caution patients during the early stages to do only 50 percent of what they feel capable of doing. It also helps to enter the process of healing with the mind-set that you are a willing, active participant, ready to bring whatever it takes to the table.
2. **The body heals on a priority basis.**
   The body has a finite amount of energy available to it at all times. As the law of energy conservation states, energy cannot be created nor be destroyed, and it can only be transferred. We already discussed this phenomenon in chapter 10, but it is so important that I want to touch on it again. Let's pretend this energy is equivalent to a $100 bill. Each function and metabolic process in your body requires a predetermined amount of energy. For example, the simple act of walking may require $5. However, if you have an injury to your right foot, such as a twisted ankle, walking may now requires $15 instead of $5. The additional $10 cannot be simply created, and it has to be transferred from other areas. This may leave every other body part and function now lacking the energy to be performed optimally. The injured part is essentially "vampiring" energy away from other parts of the body. The brain will not

allow this "energy leak" to go on fruitlessly for too long. If an injury does not heal after a while, the brain will start to ignore it.

Using the same reasoning, the nervous system will always focus most of its energy on the injury that threatens your survival the most. While CRPS may be your most painful injury, it may not be your most *life-threatening* injury. If you have heart problems, for example, these problems may be silent but ultimately prove to be more deathly. Your body, in its infinite wisdom, knows where to focus its healing energy. Conversely, as the main sight affected by CRPS begins to heal, you may feel pain somewhere new as your body is cycling through old injuries as it now has the energy freed up, which allows it to shift focus. This means that old injuries (such as disc problems) may suddenly hurt more.

In addition, my patients have frequently reported that as the limb/area affected by CRPS gets better, they will now feel the pain of CRPS elsewhere in the body for brief periods of time. This does not mean that the CRPS is spreading. It means that CRPS was already affecting other parts of your body you were just not aware of it. Pain is used by the nervous system as a fire alarm of sort. It alerts the brain to areas that require healing. You cannot get better unless your nervous system is made aware of every malfunctioning area or body part.

3. **You will lose your "pain callus."**

Healing means ups and downs, rather than smooth sailing. Some days you may feel incredibly good, and other days may plunge you back into the bowels of hell. People who suffer from daily chronic intense pain will develop what I refer to as a "pain callus." This is a protective mechanism used by the brain that prevents a massive daily leak of energy as discussed above. You cannot survive for long if you are hemorrhaging precious energy. For this reason your brain is forced to start ignoring pain to a large extent. The minute your brain unleashes your inner healing, your body will return to a state where it experiences pain the same way normal people do. For this reason, you will now experience pain differently. This means that when the pain does come back, even though it won't be worse, you will *perceive* it as more intense.

Coupled with this phenomenon is the fact that no matter how many times I tell my patients that ups and downs are to be expected and that the pain won't disappear for good after one treatment (except for a very lucky few), a part of them will still be crushed by disappointment when they have a bad day. It is one thing to hurt every day and have an uneasy acceptance of this daily pain, but to get excited and have a glimpse of heavenly normalcy and *then* to hurt again is petrifying. The first thought that will pop in your mind is, "Oh no, is the pain back? Was it too good to be true?" As time goes by and your pain goes down again and your new low pain levels become more stable, you will learn to trust your body's ability to rebound.

4. **Change is scary!**

When you picture being healthy again, I bet you never expect that feeling better may be petrifying at times. That makes no sense, right? I have observed, however, that healing is, in fact, very scary. It took me a long time to understand this phenomenon. As humans, we are naturally scared of change. Change requires our nervous system to adapt to its new circumstances, and it requires our lives to change as well. When you suffer from a chronic condition, you start to view yourself differently. Others start to view you differently too. You getting better will require those around you to get used to a new you too.

Your daily responsibilities at home change in some very practical ways. You may no longer help around the house, cook, or do your own laundry. Your relationships change also. In addition, if you have suffered from CRPS for a year or longer, you typically have been forced to change your circumstances in order to adapt. You may no longer be working. You may have given up on hobbies and traveling. You may have lost friendships and other relationships. You and your partner may have changed the way you relate to each other, as you became the dependent one and your partner the caregiver. Healing may require practical changes in your relationships. If you share children with a partner, he or she may have gotten used to being a single parent essentially and making all decisions on his or her own. Your partner may also be used to being in charge of most of the decision-making when it comes to other things, such as finances. While this may be a burden, it may also be hard to give back some of the power he or she has grown accustomed to. This does not make him or her controlling, simply human.

Getting better may leave you feeling a little bit like Rip Van Winkle, waking up to a changed world. You may have to start all over, in a sense. If you have ever observed a butterfly breaking out of its cocoon, you will know that this change has to happen very slowly. Luckily, most people will adapt after a few months and embrace life with a gratitude that can only come from literally having been to hell and back. After you return to normal life, you will always appreciate it in ways normal people will never understand. This will be a gift that you get to keep, one of the few positive things that CRPS will bring to your life.

PARTING WORDS OF WISDOM

1) **Find life rafts:** I strongly urge anyone who suffers from CRPS to find a good counselor, familiar with dealing with those in chronic pain. Both you and your partner will benefit immensely from the help of a professional as you navigate the chaotic maze that CRPS will turn your life into. CRPS tends to take no prisoners, and generally that applies to your relationship too. CRPS places immense stress on your body, your psyche, your life, and your loved ones. Do not be too proud to realize that you need professional help. Generally, you cannot expect your doctor to be your counselor also.

In addition, you will benefit immensely from any positive habits that you can bring into your life, such as meditation and talking to others who suffer from CRPS and can relate to you in a positive way. I do not advocate support groups that tend to focus on the negative aspects of CRPS. While you certainly have every reason to throw yourself a pity party, you deserve better. Remember that what you focus on expands. You may hit low points and feel the need to reach out to others and express your fears, anger, and frustration, and that is OK. However, your support group should generally add positive energy to your life.

2) **Ruthlessly cut out negative people who do not support your fight for recovery:** Unless, of course, they are family, and even then you should minimize your contact with them as much as possible. In their case, put on your invisible "Teflon" coat so all their verbal arrows just bounce off you. If you have toxic friends, acquaintances, or support groups, cut them loose. You cannot afford negativity in your life. Do not listen to anyone who tells you that you will never get better. You simply cannot afford to buy into this mind-set.

3) **Stop apologizing for being sick:** It's not your fault. All the guilt in the world will not bring your old life back, will not pay the bills, and will not take pressure off your loved ones. Guilt, in this case, is a wasted emotion, draining your energy like water into parched earth. You cannot pay guilt coins and make things better. It is a useless emotion under these circumstances, and you can better apply that wasted energy much more efficiently somewhere else.

4) **Study those who went into remission:** If you run into other CRPS sufferers in your support groups or other circles who say that they have recovered to some degree, ask them questions. Do not automatically assume that they are full of it. Friend them on social media if possible, and do not only ask them questions, but look at their posted photographs and other posts so that you may be inspired by their paths.

5) **Become your own advocate**: Your health is your responsibility. It is absolutely irresponsible to hand over your most precious possessions (your body and your health) to your doctor, blindly trusting him or her. You should research every treatment, every medication, and every supplement suggested to you. Do not just Google the official websites either, but look up, for example, "Drug X side effects." That way, you will connect with ten thousand actual people who took or are taking drug X, discussing their own experiences with it. Get into the habit of taking your pain medication only when you have to. Never let taking medications become a habit.

6) **Become a researcher:** Stay on top of your condition. Do not expect your doctor to do this for you. With the Internet at your fingertips, this is not as hard as it used to be. Try using Google Scholar when looking for the latest research. For example, just type in "Irritable Bowel Syndrome CRPS." The research is always dated. Not all articles are free, but many are. Print out relevant research, and share that with your doctor.

7) **You have the right to be supported:** Consider your condition to be a serious one. Sometimes, when so many doubt you, you may start doubting yourself. While it is good to stay positive, please do not feel the need to pretend that you feel good all the time. When you stuff all that pain down where others can't see it, you only do more damage. If people around you offer their support, accept it. Try to find others in the same boat to whom you can vent every now and then. It may be a good idea to sit down with people you are fairly close to (not just your very inner circle) and explain to them that your condition causes you to hurt every day. I tell my patients to word it something like this: "I want you to know how much our relationship means to me. I know that you care about me and my health, and I appreciate it. Generally, I am going to have pain every day. I appreciate it so much when you ask me how I am feeling, since it makes me

feel that you care. Please understand, though, that generally my good days will be very rare. It is important for me to say this to you, as I sometimes feel that people get frustrated if my answers never change. Does this make sense to you?" Most people will respond positively to this conversation, and if they don't, that is not your problem.

8) **Keep expecting to heal:** My opinion here might not be popular, but I stand firmly by it. If you decide that you will never get better and that CRPS will be your lifelong companion, the chances are that you are right. You have to keep on fighting, keep an open mind, keep researching, and keep your eyes and ears open for new developments. Like the saying goes, whether you think you can or think you can't, you are probably right.

9) **Approach your body as a unit, not a bunch of parts:** Start understanding how one part connects with another part. Develop a basic philosophy and appreciation for how the body works and how intelligent it is. Rebuild and heal it as a unit. Make sure you understand sympathetic versus parasympathetic function.

10) **Be kind to your body:** To the extent that you can, support your body with good food, good water, sunshine, and love. No one needs this more than you do. Every available speck of energy should be conserved in your case so that it can be applied to healing. You do not need to waste energy on things like unhealthy food, emotional stress, smoking, or other energy thieves.

11) **Learn how to wake up your parasympathetic nervous system:** Remember, this is your "rest and digest" nervous system. Simple things like mediation (I like Wayne Dyer's book *Getting in the Gap* to start with) or breathing exercises, if performed every day habitually, can be tremendously helpful in this regard.

12) **Try not to isolate yourself from the world:** When you need a hug, ask for one. When you are having a bad day, share that. Try to interact with your friends and loved ones as much as you can, even if it means that you are just watching a movie with them on

the couch in your PJs. Even getting some of you is still better for them than none of you at all.

13) **Give all disciplines of health care an equal shot:** I have run into this often. People often seem disappointed that I am not a medical doctor. "Oh. You're a chiropractor." Don't be a health-care snob! No matter what the letters behind their name says, it is my opinion that doctors and other professionals learn what *really* matters after they graduate, through experience and postgraduate studies. Your guide to health may not be a medical doctor or even a doctor. Research their results, and make sure that they are knowledgeable and good at what they do.

14) **Do not put up with any abusive behavior or bad treatment from a health-care professional:** If your doctor is ignorant about CRPS and unwilling to learn, fire the doctor. A good sign of this is if he or she accuses you of faking or exaggerating real pain or saying ignorant things, for example, that CRPS cannot spread or affect the GI tract. If your doctor is short, rude, dismissive, or uncaring, also fire him or her. Again, you employ your doctor, not the other way around. Doctors are not untouchable gods who may not be questioned or relieved from their employment as your caregivers. They are mortals.

Thank you for reading my book. While you and I may never meet in person, I want you to know how deeply sorry I am that CRPS happened to you or your loved one. It is a terrible condition, as close to hell on earth as one can get. However, the Force that made your body did not leave you defenseless, nor did It abandon you. That Force is inside your body now, waiting to be unleashed. Remember how immensely intelligent your body is. You were built from two cells (a sperm and an egg) into the magnificent human being that you are today. All of this required no thought from you and no medical intervention. The Force that orchestrated this miracle did not leave you to die suffering from CRPS. Others have beaten it, and so can you. Do not accept this fate.

Putting Out the Fire

I don't know what your tomorrow holds, but I do know that you must not stop seeking answers. As Albert Einstein once said, insanity is defined as doing the same thing over and over, expecting different results. I do not know if remission is in your future. What I do know is that to the best of your ability, you must not leave any stone unturned in your quest to recover. That way, when your life comes to an end one day, your loved ones will know that regardless of the outcome, you fought. Like a warrior, you fought, for that is what you are.

May the road rise up to meet you
May the wind always be at your back
May the sun shine warm upon your face,
and rains fall soft upon your fields.

—An old Irish blessing

"Don't deny the diagnosis; try to defy the verdict."

—Norman Cousins

The End

Acknowledgements

To my family, thank you for allowing me to live my passion with all your support. Thank you for all the sacrifices you didn't choose, but which you lovingly tolerate. Dad, thank you for leaving the footprints in which I could follow. Mom, thank you for the love of writing; it is one of many great things you gave to me.

To my sweet children, thoughts of helping to make this sometimes-cruel world just a little bit better inspired me to write this book. Special thanks to my little baby son, Easton, who spent many hours cramped up with a warm computer next to him before being born. I will always remember writing this while he was growing inside of me. Today, I finish it with one arm cradling his six-week old little awesome self.

Thank you to my team, without whom this would be so much harder. I know you love our patients as much as I do.

To my patients. Thank you for believing in me. Thank you for trusting me enough to bring me your proverbial broken wings, for sharing your suffering, for handing me your trust, for believing, and for still holding on to hope. You taught me much and made all of this possible.

Last but not least, I would like to thank my evil Mac on which I wrote this. You may have eaten half my book, but you did not crush me. Oh no! You taught me about seeing through things that matter and overcoming crippling disappointment. Oh, and also about external backup. You and I still have a date with a really big hammer, now that this is done…

Other Book by this Author

Taming the Beast: A Guide to Conquering Fibromyalgia

References

1. L. Van der Laan, H. ter Laak, A. Gabreels-Festen, F. Gabreels, and R. Goris, "Complex Regional Pain Syndrome type I (RSD) Pathology of Skeletal Muscle and Peripheral Nerve," *Neurology* 51, no. 1 (1998): 20–25.

2. P. Veldman, H. Reynen, I. Arntz, and R. Goris, "Signs and Symptoms of Reflex Sympathetic Dystrophy: Prospective Study of 829 Patients," *Lancet* 342 (1993): 1012–16.

3. A de Rooij, M. de Mos, M. Sturkenboom, J. Marinus, A. van den Maagdenberg, and J. van Hilten, "Familial Occurrence of Complex Regional Pain Syndrome," *European Journal of Pain* 13, no. 2 (2012): 171–77.

4. M. Pellegrino, G. Walonis, and A. Sommer, "Familial Occurrence of Primary Fibromyalgia," *Archives of Physical Medicine and Rehabilitation* 70, no. 1 (1989): 61–63.

5. S. Roizenblatt, S. Tufik, J. Goldenberg, L. Pinto, M. Hilario, and D. Feldman. "Juvenile Fibromyalgia: Clinical and Polysomnographic Aspects," *Journal of Rheumatology* 24, no. 3 (1997): 579–85.

6. C. McCabe, R. Haigh, E. Ring, P. Halligan, P. Wall, and D. Blake. "A Controlled Pilot Study of the Utility of Mirror Visual Feedback in the Treatment of CRPS (Type 1)," *British Society for Rheumatology* 42 (2003): 97–101.

7. W. Janig and R. Baron, "Complex Regional Pain Syndrome: Mystery Explained?," *The Lancet Neurology* 2 (2003): 687–97.

8. R. Alonso-Zaldivar, "Report: Health Care Costs to Account for One-fifth of U.S. Economy by 2020," *Huffington Post*, 2015.

9. R. Castro, I. Rivera, E. Struys, E. Jansen, P. Ravasco, M. Camilo, H. Blom, C. Jakobs, and I. Tavares de Almeida, "Increased Homocysteine and S-Adenosylhomocysteine Concentrations and DNA Hypomethylation in Vascular Disease," *Clinical Chemistry* 49 (2003): 1292–96.

10. P. Anderson, "Statistical Analysis: MTHFR Defects in the Chronic Fatigue Syndrome (CFS) and Fibromyalgia (FMS) Population," Available online 2012.

11. A. Inanir, S. Yigit, A. Tekcan, F. Pinarli, S. Inanir, and N. Karakus, "Angiotensin Converting Enzyme and Methylenetetrahydofolate Reductase Gene Variations in Fibromyalgia Syndrome," *Gene* 564 (2015): 188–92.

12. M. Mattson, "Methylation and Acetylation in Nervous System Development and Neurodegenerative Disorders," Laboratory of Neurosciences. National Institute on aging gerontology research center. Available online 2003.

13. M. Troen, "The Central Nervous System in Animal Models of Hyperhomocysteinemia," *Progress in Neuro-Psychopharmacology and Biological Psychiatry* 29 (2005): 1140–51.

14. M. Passatore and S. Roatta, *Influence of Sympathetic Nervous System on Sensorimotor Function: Whiplash Associated Disorders (WAD) as a Model*. Department of Neuroscience, Physiology Division, University of Torino Medical School, 2006.

15. D. Reis, D. Ruggiero, and S. Morrison, *The C1 Area of the Rostral Ventrolateral Medulla Oblongata. A Critical Brainstem Region for*

Control of Resting and Reflex Integration of Arterial Pressure (New York: Division of Neurobiology, Cornell University Medical College, 1989).

16. K. Adebove, D. Emerton, and T. Hughes, "Cervical Sympathetic Chain Dysfunction after Whiplash Injury," *Journal of the Royal Society of Medicine* 93, no. 7 (2000): 378–79.

17. J. Maleki, A. Lebel, G. Bennett, and R. Schwartzmann, "Patterns of Spread in Complex Regional Pain Syndrome, Type I (Reflex Sympathetic Dystrophy)," *Pain* 88 (2000): 259–66.

18. J. Taylor and L. Twomey, *Acute Injuries to Cervical Joints. An Autopsy Study of Neck Sprain* (Nedlands: Department of Anatomy and Human Biology, University of Western Australia, 1993).

19. M. Sasamoto, H. Chen, and S. Tsukahara, "Autonomic Nerves Containing Substance P in the Aqueous Outflow Channels and Scleral Spur of the Guinea Pig," *Japanese Journal of Ophthalmology* 43, no. 4 (1999): 272–78.

20. H. Llu, P. Mantyh, and A. Basbaum, *NMDA-receptor Regulation of Substance P Release from Primary Afferent Nociceptors* (San Francisco, CA: Departments of Anatomy and Physiology, and W. M. Keck Foundation Center for Integrative Neuroscience, University of California San Francisco, 1997).

22. S. Oke, K. Tracey, "From CNI-1493 to the Immunological Homunculus: Physiology of the Inflammatory Reflex," *Journal of Leukocite Biology* 83 (2008): 512–17.

17. B. Olshansky, H. Sabbah, P. Hauptman, and W. Colucci, "Parasympathetic Nervous System and Heart Failure, Pathophysiology and Potential

Implications for Therapy," *Contemporary Reviews in Cardiovascular Medicine* 118 (2008): 863–71.

18. K. Tracey, "Physiology and Immunology of the Cholinergic Anti-Inflammatory Pathway," *Journal of Clinical Investigation* 117 (2007): 289–96.

19. P. Mills and J. Dimsdale, "Sleep Apnea: A Model for Studying Cytokines, Sleep, and Sleep Disruption," 18 (2004): 298–303.

20. M. Maes, "The Cytokine Hypothesis of Depression: Inflammation, Oxidative and Nitrosative Stress and Leaky Gut as New Targets for Adjunctive Treatments in Depression," *Neuro Endocrinology Letters* 29, no. 3 (2008): 287–91.

21. J. Alcock, C. Maley, and C. A. Aktipis, "Is Eating Behavior Manipulated by the Gastrointestinal Microbiotica? Evolutionary Pressures and Potential Mechanisms," *Bioessays* 36 (2014): 940–49.

22. D. Hollander, "Intestinal Permeability, Leaky Gut, and Intestinal Disorders," *Current Gastroenterology Reports* 1 (1999): 410–16.

23. J. Albina and J. Reichner, "Nitric Oxide in Inflammation and Immunity," *New Horizons* 3 (1995): 46–64.

24. P. Pacher, J. S. Beckman, and L. Liaudet, "Nitric Oxide and Peroxynitrite in Health and Disease," *Physiological Reviews* 87 (2007): 315–424.

25. K. Tracey, "The Inflammatory Reflex," *Nature* 420 (2002): 853–59.

26. L. Borovikova, "Vagus Nerve Stimulation Attenuates the Systemic Inflammatory Response to Endotoxin," *Nature* 405 (2000): 458–62.

27. J. Zhang and J. An, "Cytokines, Inflammation and Pain," *International Anesthesiology Clinics* 45 (2007): 27–37.

28. J. Maleki et al., "Patterns of Spread in Complex Regional Pain Syndrome, Type I."

29. G. Vighi, "Allergy and the Gastrointestinal System," *Clinical and Experimental Immunology* 153 (2008): 3–6.

30. R. Damadian and D. Chu, "The Possible Role of Cranio-Cervical Trauma and Abnormal CSF Hydrodynamics in the Genesis of Multiple Sclerosis," *Physiological Chemistry and Physics and Medical NMR* 41 (2011): 1–17.

31. T. Buffington, "Comorbidity of Interstitial Cystitis with other Unexplained Clinical Conditions," *The Journal of Urology* 172 (2004): 1242–48.

32. M. Strittmatter, M. T. Grauer, C. Fischer, G. Hamann, K. H. Hoffmann, F. Blaes, and K. Schimrigk, "Autonomic Nervous System and Neuroendocrine Changes in Patients with Idiopathic Trigeminal Neuralgia," *Cephalalgia* 16 (1996): 476–80.

33. Y. Sterner, "Prospective Study of Trigeminal Sensibility after Whiplash Trauma," *Journal of Spinal Disorders* 14 (2001): 479–86.

34. A. Guggisberg, C. Hess, and J. Mathis, "The Significance of the Sympathetic Nervous System in the Pathophysiology of Periodic Leg Movements in Sleep," *Sleep* 30 (2007): 755–66.

35. U. Wesselmann, "Neurogenic Inflammation and Chronic Pelvic Pain," *World Journal of Urology* 19 (2001): 180–85.

36. A. Kirchner, F. Birklein, and H. Stefan, "Vagus Nerve Stimulation—A New Option for the Treatment of Chronic Pain Syndromes," *Schmerz* 15 (2001): 272–77.

37. P. Geha, M. Baliki, R. Harden, W. Bauer, T. Parrish, and A. Apkarian, "The Brain in Chronic CRPS Pain: Abnormal Gray-White Matter Interactions in Emotional and Autonomic Regions," *Neuron* 60 (2008): 570–81.

38. R. Hart, M. Martelli M, and N. Zasler, "Chronic Pain and Neuropsychological Functioning," *Neuropsychology Review* 10 (2000): 131–49.

39. B. Dick and S. Rashiq, "Disruption of Attention and Working Memory Traces in Individuals with Chronic Pain," *Anesthesia and Analgesia Journal* 104 (2007): 1223–29.

40. D. Weiner, T. Rudy, L. Morrow, J. Slaboda, and S. Lieber, "The Relationship between Pain, Neuropsychological Performance, and Physical Function in Community-dwelling Older Adults with Chronic Low Back Pain," *Pain Medication* 7 (2006): 60–70.

41. A. Oaklander, J. Rissmiller, L. Gelman, L. Zheng, Y. Chang, and R. Gott, "Evidence of Focal Small-fiber axonal Degeneration in Complex Regional Pain Syndrome-I (Reflex Sympathetic Dystrophy)," *Pain* 120 (2005): 235–43.

42. G. Correll, J. Maleki, E. Gracely, J. Muir, and R. Harbut, "Subanesthetic Ketamine Infusion Therapy: A Retrospective Analysis of a Novel Therapeutic Approach to Complex Regional Pain Syndrome," *Pain Medicine* 5 (2004): 263–75.

43. J. Farndon, "Nerve Signalling: Tracing the Wiring of Life," nobelprize.org, 2009.

44. M. Varenna, S. Adami, M. Rossini, D. Gatti, L. Idolazzi, F. Zucchi, N. Malavolta, and L. Sinigaglia, "Treatment of Complex Regional Pain Syndrome Type I with Neridronate: A Randomized, Double-blind, Placebo-controlled Study," *Rheumatology* 52 (2013): 534–42.

45. M. Rossini, O. Viapiana, B. Kalpakcioglu, R. Dhangana, D. Gatti, V. Braga, E. Fracassi, and S. Adami, "Long-term Effects of Neridronate and Its Discontinuation in Patients with Primary Hyperparathyroidism," *Calcified Tissue International* 89 (2011): 21–28.

46. V. Cartsos, S. Zhu, and A. Zavras, "Biphosphate Use and the Risk of Adverse Jaw Outcomes: A Medical Claims Study of 714,217 People," *Journal of American Dental Associates* 139 (2008): 23–30.

47. M. Ware, T. Wang, S. Shapiro, A. Robinson, T. Ducruet, T. Huynh, A. Gamsa, G. Bennett, and J. P. Collet, "Smoked Cannabis for Chronic Neuropathic Pain: A Randomized Controlled Trial," *Canadian Medical Association Journal* 182 (2010): E694–701.

48. M. Pletcher, E. Vittinghoff, R. Kalhan, J. Richman, M. Safford, S. Sidney, F. Lin, and S. Kertesz, "Association Between Marijuana Exposure and Pulmonary Function Over 20 Years," *Journal of American Medicine* 307 (2012): 173–81.

49. B. Spector, "Surface Electromyography as a Model for the Development of Standardized Procedures and Reliability Testing," *Journal of Manipulative and Physiological Therapeutics* 2 (1979): 214–22.

50. J. Cram, *Clinical EMG: Muscle Scanning for Surface Recordings* (Seattle, WA: Biofeedback Institute of Seattle, 1986).

51. P. Komi and E. Buskirk, "Reproducibility of Electromyographic Measurements with Inserted Wire Electrodes and Surface Electrodes," *Electromyography* 10 (1970): 357–67.

52. J. Hayano, Y. Sakakibara, A. Yamada, M. Yamada, S. Mukai, T. Fujinami, K. Yokoyama, Y. Watanabe, and K. Takata, "Accuracy of Assessment of Cardiac Vagal Tone by Heart Rate Variability in Normal Subjects," *Journal of American Cardiology* 67 (1991): 199–204.

53. A. Terkelsen, H. Mølgaard, J. Hansen, N. Finnerup, K. Krøner, and T. Jensen, "Heart rate Variability in Complex Regional Pain Syndrome during Rest and Mental and Orthostatic Stress," *Journal of Anesthesiology* 116 (2012): 133–46.

54. M. De Couck, R. Maréchal, S. Moorthamers, J. Van Laethem, and Y. Gidron, "Vagal Nerve Activity Predicts Overall Survival in Metastatic Pancreatic Cancer, Mediated by Inflammation," *Cancer Epidemiology* 40 (2016): 47–51.

55. M. Frisch and B. Schwartz, "The Pitfalls of Hair Analysis for Toxicants in Clinical Practice: Three Case Reports," *Environmental Health Perspective* 110 (2002): 433–36.

56. N. Cheng, "The Effects of Electric Currents on ATP Production, Protein Synthesis and Membrane Transport in Rat Skin," *Clinical Orthopedics* 171 (1982): 264–72.

57. K. Weaver, "The Content of Favorable and Unfavorable Polyunsaturated Fatty Acids Found in Commonly Eaten Fish," *Journal of American Diet* 108 (2008): 1178–85.

58. Y. Taki, H. Hashizume, Y. Sassa, H. Takeuchi, M. Asano, K. Asano, and R. Kawashima, "Breakfast Staple Types Affect Brain Gray Matter

Volume and Cognitive Function in Healthy Children," *PLos One* 5 (2010): e15213.

59. K. Oh, "Carbohydrate Intake, Glycemic Index, Glycemic Load, and Dietary Fiber in Relation to Risk of Stroke in Women," *American Journal of Epidemiology* 161 (2005): 161–69.

60. S. Liu, "Fruit and Vegetable Intake and Risk of Cardiovascular Disease: The Women's Health Study," *American Society of Clinical Nutrition* 72 (2000): 922–28.

61. J. Lampe, "Health Effects of Vegetables and Fruit: Assessing Mechanisms of Action in Human Experimental Studies," *American Society of Clinical Nutrition* 1992.

62. G. Block, B. Patterson, and A. Subar, "Fruit, Vegetables, and Cancer Prevention: A Review of the Epidemiological Evidence," *Nutrition and Cancer* 18 (1992): 1–29.

63. U. Ravnskov, "Dietary Fat Intake and Risk of Stroke: Allegations about Dietary Fat Are Unfounded," *British Medical Journal* 327 (2003): 1348.

64. J. Wang, D.G. Jackson, and G. Dahl, "The Food Dye FD&C Blue No. 1 Is a Selective Inhibitor of the ATP Release Channel Panx1," *Journal of General Practice* 141 (2013): 649–56.

65. M. Morris, "Dietary Copper and High Saturated and Trans Fat Intakes Associated with Cognitive Decline," *Journal of American Medical Association* 63 (2006): 1085–88.

66. P. Autier and S. Gandini, "Vitamin D Supplementation and Total Mortality: A Meta-analysis of Randomized Controlled Trials," *Archives of Internal Medicine Journal* 167 (2007): 1730–37.

67. Y. Sato, "Menatetrenone and Vitamin D2 with Calcium Supplements Prevent Nonvertebral Fracture in Elderly Women with Alzheimer's Disease," 2005.

68. R. Perez, W. Zuurmond, P. Bezemer, D. Kuik, A. Loenen, J. de Lange, and A. Zuidhof, "The Treatment of Complex Regional Pain Syndrome Type I with Free Radical Scavengers: A Randomized Controlled Study," *Pain* 102 (2003): 297–307.

69. M. Aviram, "Pomegranate Juice Consumption for 3 Years by Patients with Carotid Artery Stenosis Reduces Common Carotid Intima-media Thickness, Blood Pressure and LDL Oxidation," *Clinical Nutrition* 23 (2004): 423–33.

70. L. Yan, K. Fujii, J. Yao, H. Kishida, K. Hosoe, J. Sawashita, T. Takeda, M. Mori, and K. Higuchi, "Reduced Coenzyme Q10 Supplementation Decelerates Senescence in SAMP1 Mice," *Experimental Gerontology* 41 (2006): 130–40.

Printed in Great Britain
by Amazon